'I couldn't love Rafael Behr's writing more. This is a beautifully written journey through personal and political history that leads you to a wonderful place: hope. Passionate, clever, and often very funny, you couldn't wish for a more eloquent guide to the landscape of the permacrisis. But as well as being able to explain how things got broken, Behr helps you believe that they can be fixed – and that there is, meantime, a way to stay sane along the way.'
Marina Hyde

'If you want to understand what turned British politics toxic there is no better guide – or antidote.'
David Baddiel

'I'm telling you it is a must-read. Quite apart from the subject matter, Rafael Behr is such an elegant writer.'
Nigella Lawson

'A wonderful meditation on populism, nationalism, politics and truth – rich with imaginative aphorisms, alert to the most unusual connections across time and space – weaving the personal and the global – a great work of political analysis.'
Rory Stewart, *The Rest is Politics* podcast's Non-Fiction Book of the Year

'Rafael Behr's writing always illuminates even the most complicated of political chaos and this book does this and so much more: it explains our entire era and how we can bear it. Enlightening, entertaining and a delight to read.'
Hadley Freeman

'For too many of us, politics has become an exercise in anguish. And few people have absorbed and endured as much toxicity and despair as political writer Rafael Behr, who in recent years has found himself documenting a national nervous breakdown at the same time as experiencing a near-fatal cardiac crisis. The resulting book could have been solipsistic, but it's not. As Behr rehabilitates physically, he does so intellectually and politically too, producing a book which is at once hopeful, restorative, universal and true. It feels like political Prozac.'
Sathnam Sanghera, bestselling author of *Empireland*

'Fascinating and hugely enjoyable, it reassured me that I'm not going mad and any book which does that is appreciated. Wide-ranging and ludicrously readable, eminently thoughtful and sane.'
Robert Webb

'How can we still care about politics without being driven to despair or madness? This is an urgent question for citizens everywhere and Rafael Behr answers it with both passion and panache in this wonderfully engaging book. Written with all the verve and wit that make Behr one of the great stylists of contemporary journalism, this is an invigorating, illuminating and hopeful lesson in how to take politics personally.'
Fintan O'Toole, columnist at the *Irish Times* and author of *Heroic Failure: Brexit and the Politics of Pain*

'Clear and courageous, Behr stands up for freedom in a world that wants to suffocate it. And he is further distinguished by his fine style.'
Matthew Parris, columnist at *The Times*

'There are few more elegant writers about politics in the English language than Rafael Behr. With his trademark command of arresting metaphor, he probes our current democratic condition with insight, empathy and wit. The result is a book whose wisdom runs very deep.'
Jonathan Freedland, bestselling author of *The Escape Artist*

'The melding of his own near-death experience, a poignant, family history and a profound analysis of four decades of political conflict shouldn't belong in the same volume; but Rafael Behr's lucid prose makes this seem like the only way to tell the story. The most stirring riposte to political extremism and shallowness that I've read in recent years.'
Sir Trevor Phillips

'Beautifully written, interweaving the personal with the political throughout, this book reminds us why democracy matters and what it will take to preserve it.'
Noreena Hertz, economist and author of *The Lonely Century: A Call to Reconnect*

'This is what great political journalism should be like: wise, witty, tough, unflinching, honest and dare I say it, compassionate too.'
Prof Michael Ignatieff, author of _Fire and Ashes: Success and Failure in Politics_

'A sharp, informed, elegant journey through twenty-first century politics. If you're struggling to understand our political times this is the book for you. Rafael Behr is a brilliant guide to the frustrations of our political age.'
Gary Gibbon, Political Editor, Channel 4 News

'Writing to die for, insights aplenty, wisdom by the bucketload: Behr's book is a real must-read for anyone interested in the past, present and future of British politics.'
Prof Tim Bale, Professor of Politics, Queen Mary University of London

'Rafael Behr diagnoses the symptoms of the illness which has infected our discourse, and offers up an antidote that is both personal and political. The perfect prescription for anyone who has found the last few years heartbreaking.'
Matt Chorley, Times Radio

'A thoughtful, sensitive and deeply personal prescription for restoring sanity to our politics. Rafael Behr offers a heart attack survivor's guide to preventing the coronaries in British politics.'
Robert Shrimsley, chief political commentator and UK editor at large of the _Financial Times_

'It is distressingly rare to find convincing defences of liberal democracy against the twin challenges of populism and nationalism. Rafael Behr does the job perfectly.'
John Peet, Political and Brexit Editor, _The Economist_

Rafael Behr is a political journalist and broadcaster. He writes a political column for the *Guardian*. His work has also been published in *The Times*, the *Sunday Times*, the *New York Times*, the *Irish Times* and *Prospect* magazine. He is regularly a commentator on the BBC, Sky News and Times Radio. He also hosts the *Politics on the Couch* podcast. Rafael was formerly Political Editor for the *New Statesman*, chief leader writer for the *Observer*, a business writer for BBC News Online and a foreign correspondent for the *Financial Times*, based in Russia and the Baltic region.

Politics:
A Survivor's Guide

RAFAEL BEHR

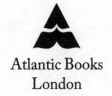

Atlantic Books
London

Published in hardback in Great Britain in 2023 by Atlantic Books,
an imprint of Atlantic Books Ltd.

10 9 8 7 6 5 4 3 2

A CIP catalogue record for this book is available from the British Library.

Hardback ISBN: 978 1 83895 504 5
E-book ISBN: 978 1 83895 505 2

Printed and bound by CPI (UK) Ltd, Croydon CR0 4YY

Atlantic Books
An imprint of Atlantic Books Ltd
Ormond House
26–27 Boswell Street
London
WC1N 3JZ

www.atlantic-books.co.uk

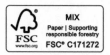

For Emily, Edie and Martha

CONTENTS

AUTHOR'S NOTE

British politics was not calm in the year when this book was written. There were three prime ministers, one of whom lasted barely six weeks in office, although she crammed a formidable volume of chaos into such a short time. I worked quickly, but events also moved fast.

Relentless political frenzy has been a boon and a challenge when writing about the health of democracy. It vindicated my choice of subject while complicating the task of capturing it in print. I had to include new evidence that supported my argument without getting swept up in a rolling carnival of ineptitude that paid no heed to my publisher's deadlines.

At some point I had to stop and send the manuscript. I shudder to imagine what new turmoil might have unfolded in the months between completion of the last draft and its publication as the volume you are now holding.

Decades of writing for daily papers and websites have ingrained in me a horror of printing something that is overtaken by breaking news and an impulse to be always revising and rewriting. But this is not a piece of journalism. The task I set myself was to understand the causes of a chronic condition, not to list every symptom.

Another journalistic foible is the tendency to privilege the recent over the significant. (That is one definition of news.) I have tried instead to maintain some distance from the daily churn of events and focus on the forces beneath them. The book is partly about the benefit of retaining that perspective. Whether I managed it isn't for me to judge.

What follows describes the evolution of turmoil, personal and political, over many years. That account should not be made obsolete by unforeseen events. But, paradoxically, the closer the narrative gets to the present, the faster it goes out of date. Facts will change, new information will come to light. The passage of time can falsify things that seemed true when I wrote them. I can't insure the text against errors of that kind, but I do apologize for them in advance.

January 2023

INTRODUCTION

HEART FAILURE

Our perspective on the past alters. Looking back, immediately in front of us is dead ground. We don't see it, and because we don't see it this means that there is no period so remote as the recent past.

Alan Bennett

(i) The widow-maker

On 31 December 2019, shortly after two o'clock in the afternoon, I put on my running kit and set off from my home in Brighton. The weather was mild for late December, but there was still a chill in the air that felt sharp in my lungs once I started breathing hard, which I did almost immediately. I trotted in the direction of the local park, roughly a kilometre from my front door, all downhill. A 45-year-old man jogging not very fast should manage the journey without stopping.

Around three quarters of the way there, I felt a familiar tightness in my lungs; a pinch that also burned. It was a sensation I had come to think of as *that chest feeling* – a syndrome associated with running that I thought was normal for middle-aged men who exercised sporadically. I had lived with it for years, carrying it ruefully as a badge of age and unfitness. When

I got back from a run, I would collapse onto the sofa clutching my chest, panting and wincing, my face flashing red and white, barely able to speak.

'Are you all right?' my wife would ask.

'Yeah . . . just . . . gimme . . . a . . . second.'

Eventually, my breathing would return to normal, and that chest feeling would subside. So when it appeared on that New Year's Eve run, I was frustrated but not alarmed. Then my chest exploded. First, a detonation in my ribs. Then waves of hot pain came streaming out from behind my lungs, like lava from a volcano. Molten agony seared up and over my left shoulder, down my arm to the tips of my fingers. I stopped running.

Along with the burn, there came a crumpling constriction, as if my chest was trying to fold itself into a smaller person. Also, a wave of nausea that leaked out from my body and soured everything I could see. The sky darkened and curled at the edges, like paper on a fire. I felt drenched in impending doom; an all-encompassing state of ill-being. The air tasted ominous. It took me around 30 seconds of weighing the evidence before deciding to go home. On one hand (the left one, in particular), I appeared to be experiencing exactly the sort of things you might expect while suffering a massive heart attack. But on the other hand, that was the sort of thing that only happened to other people.

Besides, we had old friends coming for dinner. I was looking forward to a fun evening. It would be preposterous to have a heart attack now. I had already prepared the salmon.

Then I remembered Eric Rink.

One Sunday morning in Cape Town, 12 years before I was born, Eric Rink had gone to play golf, as he often did at the weekend. He always returned in time for lunch. But on this particular Sunday, lunch went cold on the table. Eric never came home. His heart had stopped. He was 45 years old. His daughter, my mother, was 14 at the time.

My maternal grandfather's absence had always been a vague presence in my life – a story only half told. I knew that he had been an aerial photographer in the Second World War, taking reconnaissance pictures of bomb sites; that he was born Eliyahu Rinkunsky into the large Jewish population of Lithuania; that the surname had been truncated by a South African immigration official when the family emigrated in the 1920s.

The name Eric was chosen later. The rebrand was suggested by his wife, Dina, my grandmother, after the war, when Ely (as he continued to be known to family) set up a commercial photography studio. He had a blue Ford Prefect with 'Eric Rink Portrait Studios' painted down the side in red. He and my mother had been close. He had sometimes taken her to the studio and taught her how to develop prints in the darkroom. I knew that she was the same age as my own daughter when she lost him. It was enough information to steer me into a U-turn and send me loping and staggering back up the hill towards home. I remembered that heart attacks were exactly the sort of thing that sometimes happened to middle-aged men like me.

My wife drove me to the hospital. I pressed my back hard into the passenger seat and gripped the door handle. I wound down the window, hunting the oxygen that refused to enter my lungs. We stopped at a red light. Ambulances are allowed to ignore these, I said, unhelpfully.

The hospital was no more than 15 minutes away. I told myself I was not going to die because I would soon be in front of a doctor and medical science had come a long way since my grandfather's day. It occurred to me that there is a moment when every parent sees their children for the last time, and that mine might already have passed that morning. I didn't remember what I had said. It wasn't goodbye.

There are no good heart attacks, but some are worse than others. Mine was a major obstruction to the left anterior descending artery, the main pipe supplying the left ventricle, which pumps oxygenating blood to the vital organs of the body. Somewhere inside that pipe was a plaque caused by cholesterol deposits that had built up over years – a fatberg. It split open as I was running down the road and clogged the artery. My blood cells then tried to be useful and formed a clot at the site of the rupture, which compounded the blockage. If you are lucky, a heart attack is a traffic jam on one of the B roads of the arterial network. By the time I reached the hospital, I had blocked both carriageways of the M25.

Old-school cardiologists call it 'the widow-maker'. The longer you leave it, the higher the risk of ventricular fibrillation, where the heart muscle goes into spasm and, if not treated quickly, stops beating altogether. You then need someone to sit on top of you compressing your chest until an electrical defibrillator can be applied. Two paddles, administering up to 1,000 volts, can jump-start the heart back into a steady rhythm.

We arrived at the hospital. I got out of the car while it was still moving and loped into A&E. I saw the reception window up ahead and thought about how best to communicate my predicament. I collapsed onto the floor, which did the job. I was soon on a bed moving down corridors.

The diagnosis didn't take long.

Doctor (hurriedly): Have you taken any illegal drugs, Mr Behr?

Me (defensively): What, ever?

Doctor: Today, in the past 24 hours.

Me: Oh, right. No.

Doctor: Do you know of any family history of heart disease?

Me: Yes. Both sides.

Cardiac calamity had been advancing in a pincer movement down the generations towards me. It wasn't just Eric Rink. My paternal grandfather had also died from a heart attack. My dad had recently needed a triple bypass.

'Next time, call an ambulance,' the doctor said.

Pro tip, I thought, but I'm not planning on making this a regular gig.

I was taken to the coldest room on earth. I later learned that the temperature had to be kept low because the high-tech machines involved in scanning and probing a heart can over-heat. I was still in my running kit and felt underdressed for the occasion. That, combined with the general state of shock and failing blood circulation, caused one side of my body to shake violently. The other side would have joined in, but it was held down by surgeons and nurses trying to insert a catheter through a small incision in my wrist.

Angioplasty is a marvel of science. The catheter is passed up the arm, over the shoulder and into the heart. Dye is injected, which shows up on a scan, revealing the location of the pro-blem. I could see it on the screen, clouds of inky reflux bouncing back from the place where the blood wasn't flowing properly.

Once the blockage is located, it can be forced open again with stents – tiny inflatable tubes that reinforce the artery wall. I was conscious through all of this but full of morphine – full in the sense that I had reached the safe limit, not in the sense of sated. I asked for more, but was told I had maxed out.

The drugs did strange things to my sense of time. It felt as if the whole thing passed in a few minutes, but some of those minutes took years. The catheter smooshes open the artery, but the inflation of the stent temporarily re-blocks it. That feels like starting the heart attack from the beginning again. Then the balloon inside the stent is withdrawn, and blood can rush through. At that point, every cell of my body gave a little cheer, like a nation of drought-stricken farmers celebrating the first drops of rain on parched fields. When the surgeon loaded up a second stent, I braced myself. I didn't want the nice cool rain feeling to stop.

'Could you just give me a moment?' I asked.

He shook his head. 'Time is very much of the essence here, Mr Behr.'

By early evening, I was lying in a hospital bed, pale, weak, with a lingering pain in my chest but otherwise feeling marvellous. My mood overshot relief and landed somewhere in exuberant conviviality. I tried to joke with the nurses, but the morphine had me less than coherent. Also, cardiac emergency wards aren't very funny places. I sent upbeat messages to friends and family explaining where I was and how I had got there, as if dispatching postcards from an exotic holiday. I told work I'd be back at my keyboard soon.

Psychologists call it survivor elation. My body was physically debilitated but also hyper-alert from shock and adrenaline.

When people came to visit, they found my joviality discon-certing, given how terrible I looked. It was a matter of alternate perspectives; different ways of registering the same information. They saw the old me, diminished by a brush with mortality. All I could feel was the upside of still being alive.

Then the consultant came round and explained that my heart, having been starved of oxygen, was operating at around a fifth of normal capacity. An unknown portion of the damaged muscle was merely stunned and would wake up in time. Mean-while, I was in a condition technically classified as heart failure – the organ wasn't up to the job. It could pump enough to get me across a room, but not far; not up a flight of stairs.

The prognosis wasn't too bad. I was relatively young for a cardiac patient. I didn't feel very young. I asked the doctor if events of this magnitude were common in people my age. He said: 'You were unlucky to have a heart attack that big so young, but lucky to be young enough to survive a heart attack that big.' Neat, I thought.

A cardiac nurse talked me through the rules once I was allowed to go home: build up activity gradually; listen to your body; don't be afraid to move around but don't push your luck; no heavy lifting. And above all, avoid stress.

What did I do for a living? Journalism.

What did I write about? Politics. Oh, how interesting. Was that stressful?

(ii) Attack of the Furies

In the parliamentary press gallery, where I worked, we had joked about 'Brexit Derangement Syndrome'. It was an affliction among MPs who had previously seemed quite balanced but lost all sense of perspective working themselves into hysterical lathers over the politics of leaving the European Union. It erupted in the Commons chamber from time to time but was more pronounced on social media, inflamed by a million amateur demagogues.

People who had voted for Brexit in the 2016 referendum were frustrated that it wasn't happening faster. People who thought Brexit would be a disaster found vindication in the bungled implementation. The righteous indignation of each side stoked the other's resentment, whipping politics into a frenzy of rage and despair.

British politics had been in febrile campaign mode for years. It started with the 2014 referendum on Scottish independence. Then there was a general election in 2015, followed by an exceptionally fissile Labour leadership contest, triggering a protracted civil war on the left over the wisdom of keeping Jeremy Corbyn as leader. Then came the Brexit plebiscite, followed by a Tory leadership contest, which made Theresa May prime minister. Then a general election in 2017. The level of public enthusiasm for yet another ballot, promising more heated rhetoric, more uncertainty, was communicated by Brenda from Bristol, a middle-aged woman who was accosted by a BBC news crew on the day the election was called and asked what she made of it:

'You're joking. What? Another one. Honestly. I can't stand this. There's too much politics going on at the moment.'

There was too much politics, but there was about to be a whole lot more. The election produced a hung parliament. Corbyn did much better than his critics predicted, but still lost – a result that further aggravated Labour's internecine strife. May clung on to power, but without authority, having squandered her parliamentary majority.

There followed two nerve-shredding years of legislative deadlock over Brexit. The wheels of political debate were spinning frictionlessly without propelling the argument or the country forwards. A lot of people were radicalized in the process. I had been a committed Remainer in 2016. Part of that choice was patriotism. I liked Britain and didn't want it to undergo what I saw as pointless damage. I was also attached to the founding idea of the European Union. I believed in political integration as the antidote to the bloodthirsty nationalism that had once made the continent so unsafe for my grandparents that they had fled to another hemisphere.

It pained me to lose the argument for Britain's alignment with that ideal, but not as much as it hurt when the winners turned vindictive in their victory, referring to the losers as quislings and traitors. When May called the 2017 election, the front page of the *Daily Mail* had urged her to 'crush the saboteurs'.

Like many Remainers, I had so much anger sloshing around inside me that there wasn't a lot of room for sympathy with the other side. The rational part of me recognized a journalistic duty to see things from their point of view. I knew that Euroscepticism had deep cultural roots and that the vote had given expression to social and economic grievances that had been brewing for decades. I could see how irritating it must have been, having cast a ballot for drastic change, to find the country bogged down in pernickety parliamentary wrangling over the small print. On a calm day, I could appreciate how arrogant and undemocratic it looked to Leavers when

Remainers insisted on re-asking the question in order to solicit a better answer. Our anger was making them angrier, which was fuelling the nationalistic rhetoric that was making us fearful and less inclined to compromise.

No one was satisfied. But some of us were suffering in metric units and some were measuring their outrage in imperial yards. The tragedy was that we couldn't find a formula to convert one into the other.

I also felt homeless in Britain's party system. I had always been a Labour voter, but that allegiance was broken by an epidemic of anti-Semitism under Corbyn. Jewish Labour MPs were hounded out of the party and the leader didn't lift a finger to protect them. His fingers were busy wagging at journalists for querying his record of comradeship with terrorist sympathizers and Holocaust deniers. He was a magnet for every crank who imagined Jews pulling the strings behind the scenes of media and government.

Then the Tories elected Boris Johnson as their leader, a man as unsuitable to be prime minister as Corbyn, but for different reasons. As the 2019 election loomed, I wanted them both to lose. I imagined them colliding and cancelling each other out, like something from a science fiction movie: two particles fired into each other from opposite ends of the political spectrum head on, causing both candidates to be vaporized; a flash, a shock wave and then an eerie calm and normal politics restored. But the British electoral system didn't work like that. Normal was not an option.

I started to feel 'that chest feeling' more often. I drank too much and put on weight. In photos from that time I look puffy, a greener shade of pale. It was not the first time I had experienced work-related stress, but it was the first time I was conscious of it infusing every part of my body, stalking me, interfering with my sleep and distracting me from my family.

I failed to enforce any boundary between work and life. There was a toxic substance flowing through Westminster and it was my job to filter and siphon and analyse it, but I didn't observe good laboratory discipline. I carried it in my pocket, brought it home, spilled it on myself. My phone was the leaky vessel, dripping poison into every room. It was the last thing I saw at night and the first thing I reached for in the morning. I was spending too much time on Twitter, keeping the furnace of my anger stoked.

I was consumed by a twitchy lassitude, pulling me in opposite directions. If I was in the car and politics came on the radio, I wanted to turn it up and also turn it off. As a political columnist for a national newspaper, I felt a professional duty to throw myself into the debate. As a citizen, I felt a self-preserving instinct to pull away and hide.

The more I cared about politics, the worse I was as a husband and father. I was short-tempered, prickly, unrespon-sive. I shouted at my children and zoned out of conversations with my wife. I was present in the room and emotionally absent. I could be sitting at the table eating dinner while mentally pacing the room, knotted in agitation, turning political argu-ments over in my head.

It was an emotional vortex that fed upon itself, raging against the despondency it induced. And always there was the undertow of foreboding and a compulsion to withdraw. The Israeli writer David Grossman has called it 'a clenching of the soul'.

Politics didn't cause my heart attack. I did that myself, heaping pastries and cigarettes on top of a genetic predisposition to cardiovascular disease. But stress didn't help. By the end of 2019, when Johnson won his landslide election victory, I was furious at the state of British politics and furious *with* British politics for the state it had put me in.

I had many conversations with friends and colleagues in Westminster and beyond who felt the same. I knew journalists, MPs, civil servants, Commons clerks and special advisers who had suffered physical and mental health problems – depression, breakdowns, substance abuse, chronic anxiety – which they attributed to the furious mess of British politics. Many quit because the atmosphere was too toxic.

In ancient Greek mythology, the Furies were vengeful goddesses, progeny of darkness who hounded their victims into madness. I'm not sure what we all did to deserve that fate. Complacency was our original sin. We had not thought British politics could get so bleak, and when it felt as if the whole edifice was tipping into an abyss, we had no idea how far we could fall. History offered horrific worst-case scenarios to contemplate in the event of democracy breaking down. It was hysterical to think we were on that trajectory but irresponsible to rule it out as a possibility.

(iii) Permacrisis

'We still don't know much about this virus,' the consultant told me. 'Be careful. You could do without it.' It was a routine cardiology appointment at a time when nothing felt routine. Brexit had been swept out of the news by the novel coronavirus that had already marauded across Europe and was now infecting people in Britain. The disease was reported to be especially menacing to older people and anyone with underlying health problems. I wasn't sure whether 45 plus a dodgy ticker put me in the vulnerable category.

The doctor explained that my body was still battered and traumatized by the loss of oxygen when the artery had been blocked. 'Think of yourself as more like 55 to 60,' he told me. In the hours between the first explosive convulsion in my chest and the stents going in, I had burned through a decade's supply of heart.

In the years that followed, it felt as if the whole country experienced a trauma of accelerated ageing. The pandemic lockdowns were disorienting and also made time seem strangely elastic. It reminded me of morphine – hours lasting years, while months disappeared in seconds. The longer it went on, the clearer it became that whatever we had once thought of as 'normal' politics was consigned to history.

There was a moment when it seemed that some of the divisions might be healing. The partisan clamour of the previous years was replaced by a palpable craving for solidarity, expressed in the ritual of doorstep applause for health workers every Thursday evening. But that spirit quickly dissipated as the ordeal went on. The toll of the pandemic in terms of economic resilience and mortality rates was uneven. The virus inflamed pre-existing social morbidities. It also inflamed culture wars, the diligent and disobedient wrangling over lockdown rules and vaccines. Boris Johnson's popularity peaked when the disease nearly killed him, and then cratered when it turned out the rules imposed on the nation had been serially ignored in Downing Street.

Johnson's short but unruly period of government brought a different kind of temporal distortion. Scandal and confusion tumbled out of Downing Street so fast, it lapped the normal news cycle. One drama was not over before the next one began. Monday's outrage blurred into Tuesday's blunder, compounded by Wednesday's sordid misdemeanour, lost amid Thursday's provocation, triggering Friday's backlash. Seven days in Johnson time aged politics by more than a week.

The mood was captured by a caller to a radio phone-in after some new revelation connected to the 'Partygate' scandal that ultimately led to Johnson being ousted. I didn't catch the despondent citizen's name, but I wrote down what he said because it tallied so neatly with what I kept hearing all around me. 'I don't care any more. And I'm angry with myself for not caring any more, because I know it really does matter.'

In February 2022, Russia invaded Ukraine and shook European politics to its foundations. It was territorial aggression of a kind that had not been seen on the continent since 1945, and conceived by Vladimir Putin as a challenge to the institutions and rules of a global order that had risen from the ashes of the Second World War. It also had a second front – a war of economic attrition against Western governments that relied on Russian oil and gas exports. The pandemic was pushed aside by a cost-of-living crisis just as COVID had once submerged Brexit, which was still there in the background, an open wound poorly dressed on the body politic. Boris Johnson's government unravelled, to be replaced by Liz Truss's administration, which imploded. Britain has changed prime minister four times since the Brexit referendum – as many times as it did in the preceding thirty years.

Each crisis compounded the one before until they merged into one constant state of permacrisis. During this time of frenetic volatility, I returned to work. Slowly at first, engaging gingerly with politics, unsure whether I even wanted to go there. It felt like working as a cartographer in the middle of an earthquake, where the ground you want to map is moving and the landmarks you note are at constant risk of tumbling down.

In those conditions I found it hard to keep things in perspective. How bad was it compared to previous periods of historical disturbance? How should I judge the health of British democracy – against an ideal of how a perfect system would work or relative to other countries that were in an even worse state? How much consolation should I take from a government that was merely incompetent and self-serving when there was murderous tyranny abroad?

When events pile shock upon shock, it can be hard to *stay* shocked while also staying sane. We need to adapt to the changing shape of reality, resisting the temptations of retreat into nostalgia and disengagement. But adaptation opens the trap of normalization, where the unacceptable is rebranded as inevitable. Anger is a rational response to bad government and an ingredient in democracy. It stimulates taste for change and is a spur against apathy. But that mechanism requires confidence that the system will respond. The most toxic state is the fusion of fury and despondency, when it feels that the democratic process itself has become the engine of grievance and dis-harmony. In that doom loop of rage I came to fear elections for the rancour they might spread, when I should have cherished them as opportunities for renewal.

I was mindful of the years I had spent in denial, on both a personal and political level. I had been running with angina, stopping periodically to recover my breath, without considering the systemic obstruction building in my arteries. I had been cruising through Westminster, imagining that the politics I had known all my adult life would determine the pace and ethical parameters of politics in perpetuity.

Eric Rink, the grandfather who had died suddenly of a heart attack in 1962, had shaken me out of denial when part of me wanted to plod on through the chest pain, hoping it might subside. I turned to him again.

There aren't many pictures. He was a photographer, more likely to be holding the camera. One of the only prints I have shows him and his two brothers on the day they were demobilized after the Second World War. He had served in the South African Air Force, attached then to the British RAF, taking reconnaissance pictures. He was later haunted by the thought of images he had developed setting targets for bombs. From the stories my mother tells, it seems likely he suffered from undiagnosed post-traumatic stress.

In the photograph, you see impatience for civilian clothes tugging at the young brothers' uniforms. Their weary-eyed smiles rhyme with their crooked berets. Ely was the eldest. He had supported his younger brothers since they were children. Their father had died suddenly not long after their emigration – a heart attack. Ely was 14 years old.

I looked at that picture a lot. It became a meditation on the forces that connect people – the bonds of shared history, blood, identity and experience. This man's childhood flight from anti-Semitism in Lithuania had somehow landed me in Britain.

I found it comforting to find familiar traces in my grandfather's features: not an uncanny likeness, but unmistakable; something in the line of the chin, the nose. Also the heart. Eric Rink had nudged me to the hospital. He looked out from the photo, asking me what I planned to do now that, unlike him, I had survived.

(iv) What this book is and what it isn't about

In *Unreliable Memoirs*, Clive James wrote that 'to wait until reminiscence is justified by achievement might mean to wait forever'. This is not a memoir, but it is as much about me as anything else, apart from politics. If I had made achievement the threshold for publication, it would surely never have been written. It is unreliable to the extent that it is deliberately subjective. I have been writing about politics for more than 25 years, and have tried in that time to achieve some analytical detachment. But what appears in my newspaper column is inevitably coloured by background and personal experience. The world as I see it gets filtered through lenses of culture, history, identity. This book is about those filters – what they magnify, how they distort – as much as politics itself.

It was conceived in convalescence and in hiding from COVID. I knew that before I went back to work, I would have to learn new ways of looking at politics. I wanted to re-engage without getting enraged. That was a personal quest before it evolved into an attempt to say things of interest to anyone else. Only after conversations with enough people from different backgrounds and with different party allegiances did I start to feel confident in extrapolating from my experience to reach broader conclusions about the state of politics.

I was wary of aggrandizing a liberal whinge into a national syndrome. Or worse, there was a danger of over-diagnosing a chronic ailment where really there was just a bout of electoral indigestion from swallowing too many defeats.

How to disentangle banal dismay at being on the losing side of an argument from legitimate concern over the health of democracy? How absolute is the duty to be reconciled to bad ideas and rotten leaders if enough people have voted for them? What if those ideas and leaders undermine democracy itself? And who will judge if they do?

These are the questions I asked myself as I nursed a limping heart back to a more robust beat.

There is some elision from the first person singular to plural – what *I* think and feel blurs into what *we* face as a country. That is a big leap between small words. If it doesn't feel justified, I hope the overreach still points in a useful direction. I don't expect a reader to share my view on everything. I limit my ambition to the offer of company that might be agreeable even when we disagree.

To organize material that threatened to sprawl in every direction at once, I have given the story a beginning, a middle and an end. Each section is anchored in a phase of my own engagement with politics, but the chapters are linked more by theme than chronology.

Part One is about origins and belonging – what it means to feel connected to a country through politics; the anguish and causes of disconnection.

Part Two begins in Russia, where I was a foreign correspondent, and applies some of the lessons I learned there about how a democracy is meant to work; lessons acquired by watching one fail. From Russia, I return to British politics, polarized and carved into culture-war trenches.

Part Three is based in Westminster and charts a revolution that succeeded by exploiting huge reserves of public discontent while doomed never to satisfy those grievances. The concluding section is an attempt to put some of the observations from the previous parts into some broader global and historical perspective.

Any book steeped in lament for the health of democracy must acknowledge how often throughout history similar complaints have been made that look overwrought in hindsight. The long view of human civilization contains more grounds to believe in progress than it gives cause for panic. But the scale of current volatility militates against complacency. In my conclusions, I have tried to find a place of equilibrium between alarm and reassurance.

History doesn't naturally punctuate itself with full stops and neat paragraphs, but authors have deadlines. Mine dictated the point beyond which new developments could no longer be included in the narrative. Since most of the book is about history and trends, the absence of breaking news should not, I hope, undermine my conclusions. If recent precedent is a guide, politics will have taken dramatic turns between me writing this sentence and you reading it. I can't predict the backdrop against which the analysis in these pages will be received. I can only ask for indulgence where new facts have superseded my observations. I hope that all the years of political journalism stuffed into this book make a cushion of judgement sufficient to withstand the inevitable assault by events.

What do I mean by engagement with politics? Something more than just turning up at election time but distinct from active involvement via membership of parties and campaigns. I have great respect for people who back up their beliefs with activism. Democratic politics couldn't function without the civic spirit of volunteers who canvass for candidates, stuff envelopes, knock on doors and attend meetings in front rooms and chilly church halls. They often get a bad press as maniacs and obsessives. Some are. Mostly, in my experience, they are decent, fair-minded, principled citizens, doing a vital service for society.

But a healthy democracy also needs people in the middle, neither activist nor apathetic; engaged, but not fully immersed. The most committed participants tend not to be swing voters. Activists don't often change their allegiances. Power changes hands in free elections because of currents and trends in the broad stratum of society that cares enough about politics to follow the news, while also going about life, neither frantic to hear every latest Westminster development nor repelled by dread of what it will be. That middle tier of reasonable civic engagement is the segment I fear is being depleted and demoralized by our state of permacrisis. That is where the epidemic of rage threatens to hollow out democracy.

I cannot claim to have covered the full extent of the challenge, let alone solved it. I am sorry for all the omissions and simplifications. I could list some of them up front, but I'm too embarrassed. Large tracts of political terrain are not covered. I had to draw limits somewhere. I stuck to the narrow plot of my own experience, painfully aware that beyond lies a sweeping prairie of ignorance. I don't think my choice of material is wildly idiosyncratic, but it is personal, which might be the same thing.*

This is a book about the way a healthy democracy should connect people to each other and to the place they call home. It is about the toxic politics that disrupt and reverse that process. It is about failures at the heart of democracy, written on a journey of cardiac rehabilitation.

The world as I knew it was turned upside down by political crisis and medical emergency that happened to coincide. It would be a solipsistic fallacy to conflate the two. I briefly considered an epic allegory of heart disease in the body politic, connecting failures of political function in a democracy to the circulation of blood around vital organs, and so on. I couldn't sustain it, so I won't labour the metaphor any further. But there was therapeutic purpose to writing this book. If I was ever to resume journalism, I needed to tease out the personal, historical and cultural threads from the knot of political rage in my heart.

The result of that diagnostic disentanglement follows, in case anyone else should find it useful.

---

* I use footnotes in the text to make comments aside, like this one, not for references and sources. There are too many of those and they would clutter the text if identified by this method. There is instead a bibliography at the end.

Part One

EXILE

CHAPTER 1

THE OLD COUNTRY

Motherlands are castles made of glass. In order to leave them, you have to break something — a wall, a social convention, a cultural norm, a psychological barrier, a heart. What you have broken will haunt you. To be an émigré, therefore, means to forever bear shards of glass in your pockets. It is easy to forget they are there, light and minuscule as they are, and go on with your life, your little ambitions and important plans, but at the slightest contact the shards will remind you of their presence. They will cut you deep.

Elif Shafak

(i) Homeland insecurity

The little Lithuanian town of Linkuva, around 170 kilometres north of Vilnius, was uncertain about its Jewish past. The first person I asked, a woman at the bus station, was terse. 'No one here knows anything.' It sounded like a rebuke. 'No one remembers anything.' Many of the people I met walking into the centre of town didn't want to speak at all.

Sometimes curiosity overcame suspicion. Foreign tourists don't go to Linkuva, and visiting Lithuanians wouldn't start asking about Jews. Some people had no idea what I was talking about. Others had heard tell of a thriving community, once upon a time, but couldn't explain its disappearance.

After a succession of blank looks and sullen rejections, I finally met someone chatty. Danite was a middle-aged woman with a trapezoid frame and a silver-capped, nicotine-stained smile. She pointed out a yellow brick building set around 20 metres back from the town square. It had once been a synagogue. After the Second World War, it was converted to a cinema. When the Soviet Union collapsed and Lithuania gained its independence, the cinema fell into disuse and, judging by the smell, now served as a public toilet for people of all faiths and none.

Danite explained that many of the brick buildings in the centre of town had been the properties of Jewish tradesmen. They had been the urban middle class. The rest of the houses were wood. 'There used to be lots of Jews here,' she told me confidently, although she would have been too young to remember them. 'But they all went away. Or they got killed.'

She told me where to find the Jewish cemetery on the road out of town and drew me a map. It was easily missed, although there was a small sign in Lithuanian and Hebrew. The lopsided, broken gravestones were overgrown with weeds. Their pale grey mottled faces were barely visible from the road. There was no boundary where the grassy roadside verge ended and the cemetery began, just a crop of fractured memorials that seemed to get more numerous the longer I stared at the field and my eyes got accustomed to their camouflage. It felt like they were emerging to meet me, wary creatures intuiting that I posed no threat.

I examined a few of the headstones, but the inscriptions were badly weathered and my Hebrew, also eroded by time, wouldn't have been up to deciphering them anyway. I took some pictures with an old-style analogue camera. This was 2001, before smartphones.

When I was growing up in London, we had a stash of old sepia photographs dating back to the first decade of the twentieth century, taken in or around Linkuva. One shows a *cheder* class, a group of around 30 Jewish schoolchildren with a couple of their teachers. The children mostly appear bored, or maybe resentful at being made to sit still. They are outside a rickety-looking wooden building that is presumably the school house. The boys all have their heads covered with flat caps. One, looking younger and more alarmed than insolent, has a badge of some sort on his cap. What it designated is unknown. He is Jacob Behr, my father's father. The picture is thought to be from around 1906. Six years later, Jacob – Jack, as he would later be known – moved with his parents and a cousin to South Africa. Other cousins stayed in Lithuania.

One was Bertha Gilman – Baska to her family. We have a couple of photographs of her, too. In one, she is maybe three or four years old, fair-haired, sitting on a simple wooden chair set on the hard ground. In another picture, dated 1923, Baska is a young woman, standing for a formal portrait. She wears a long plain dark dress; her hair has turned darker too. She has a black bow or scarf tied into her hair, falling down over her shoulder. There is an inscription in Yiddish on the back, written to my grandfather and his parents. The translation:

When you take this picture in hand may you remind yourself
of the face, which was at one time well known to you, and
may you remember your relative who is over the sea, and

may you think happily of a time when we can be together. As a reminder of your dear niece and cousin.

The record goes silent after that.

The road out of Linkuva past the cemetery leads to Pashvitinys, another small town that was home to my paternal grandmother's side of the family (they called it Pashvitin). And there I stood, 27 years of age, roughly a hundred years after my great-grandparents had left, in a meadow somewhere between their home towns, staring at illegible tombstones that might have belonged to some distant family member but probably didn't. I waited solemnly for a few minutes, long enough to justify the journey to myself, reaching for some transcendental connection to the place, not feeling much more than the brush of gnats against my arms. What was Linkuva to me? A place in a story I had been told about a land we once came from called Lithuania; a point of origin in family folklore. But when I foraged for roots on the outskirts of the town, I found nothing to hold on to.

Deracinated. Literally it means uprooted. Britain was my home. But did I think of it as my home*land*? The word implies ancestral connection, although less explicitly than 'motherland' and 'fatherland'. Those terms seemed to me atavistic as well as archaic. They spoke of intimate bloodlines in a way that I associated with demagoguery and war.

As for patriotism, it was something I was still discovering in myself. I was intensifying fondness for the place I grew up by the reliable method of absence abroad. Even then, I found it easiest to be proud of British culture when it was squeamish about effusive displays of national pride, self-deprecating, understated. Asked to name the quality of Britishness I most admired, I would probably have identified the ironic humour that can't itemize national greatness without wanting to mock the pomposity of the exercise. And nationalism? I thought of it as an antique doctrine from previous centuries, a crude instrument that people had once used to dig their independence out from under foreign domination.

Nationalism was a big part of politics in Lithuania at that time, as it was in neighbouring Latvia and Estonia. The three Baltic states had only recently broken free from the Soviet Union. The engine of their liberation had been defiant assertion of national cultures – folk songs and stories in the native tongue – stubbornly preserved through decades of forced Russification.

I was there as a correspondent for the *Financial Times*, my first overseas posting, awarded to a rookie reporter on the basis that big stories rarely came out of such small countries. When the Baltic states had stood heroically against Kremlin crack-downs in the late 1980s, they had briefly felt like the centre of the world. They were the loose thread that pulled at the edge of Soviet power and unravelled the whole shoddy weave.

It was a much more slow-moving story by the time I got there a decade later. When I told people I was heading off to the Baltic, they would congratulate me for being so intrepid but wondered whether I would be safe. It usually turned out they thought I had said Balkans. They thought I was going to Europe's most notorious crucible of armed national vendettas.

Phonetic similarity wasn't the only point the two regions had in common. In the mid nineties, when civil war was ripping apart countries of the former Yugoslavia, there was some speculation among Western analysts that inter-ethnic grievances could also turn violent in the Baltic states. The fear was that communist rule had bottled a load of nationalist rage that would spill blood wherever it was uncorked. But it didn't happen. The Baltic transition to democracy was not effortless, but nor was it botched. A lot of the success was down to the twin prospects of European Union and NATO membership. That was what I spent most of my time covering as a journalist. Britain was an enthusiastic sponsor of EU enlargement to include former Warsaw Pact countries. I saw at ground level how the European project incentivized democratic reform and embedded the rule of law in places where many worse trajectories looked plausible. It was a bureaucratic miracle, which is to say it was a wonderful thing that was boring to write about as a journalist. I was happy for the Baltics that their politics were becoming more boring to the outside world.

Boring was good. Boring meant nationalist ferment subsiding.

Post-Soviet tension didn't dissipate overnight. The trickiest issue – and one where the EU and NATO leaned on nationalistic governments to adopt more liberal policies* – was citizenship rights for local Russians. There were millions of them. To many Balts, the Russians were ethnic jetsam deposited on their land when the Soviet tide rolled back eastwards. Some had family roots in the region going back generations, but most were there as a consequence of Kremlin policies that used migration of the Soviet Union's various ethnicities as an instrument of political control. Russians were deployed as demographic weapons in

---

* The situation was slightly different between the three Baltic states. I spilled a lot of ink and spent many hours of argument over the rights and wrongs of citizenship laws. It's a long and intricate story for which there isn't space here. I apologize to any Baltic readers who take issue with the briskness of my précis.

places that were thought to harbour congenital disloyalty. Sovietization, by means of Russification, was a way to suffocate 'bourgeois nationalism'.

The Baltics were especially suspect. They had been absorbed later into the Union than most Soviet republics. They had broken away from the Russian Empire amid the chaos, mud and blood of the Bolshevik Revolution and the First World War. They were independent for a couple of decades before being recaptured by Stalin as part of the territorial carve-up agreed with Hitler in 1939, formalized as the Molotov–Ribbentrop pact.*

Occupation by the Red Army was a national calamity for Lithuanians, Latvians and Estonians. Their interwar governments had started out democratic, but tilted fascist in the thirties. When Hitler did the double-cross on Stalin and the armies of the Third Reich marched east across the Baltic, many locals welcomed them as liberators. They had nothing to fear from Nazi race policies, which ranked Balts above Slavs. And, of course, much higher than Jews.

On 28 June 1941, the Germans arrived in Linkuva. Its Jewish population, depleted by years of emigration, was topped up by refugees fleeing the Nazi advance. The total was somewhere around 1,000. There is no definitive account of what happened next, but according to the testimony of the few survivors and witnesses, the Jews were rounded up by local Lithuanian

---

* That deal, named after the Soviet and Nazi foreign ministers, is more famous in Britain for partitioning Poland and starting the Second World War. In Russia, a veil is drawn over complicity with the Nazis. The national cult of military heroism focuses on 'the Great Patriotic War' that started two years later, when Hitler marched on Moscow.

police and accomplices, acting partly on orders from German commanders but made thorough in their work by native anti-Semitism. The men and women were separated, locked in local barns and warehouses that had belonged to Jewish enterprises. Over the following days, the stronger prisoners were made to dig mass graves in the nearby forest. Then all were shot. Among them Baska Gilman and an unknown number of my other relatives.

(ii) Concentric circles

When I was eight years old and needed to write my name and address, I would include as many elements as I could, expanding the sphere of reference as wide as imagination would stretch:

Rafael Behr
81 Gordon Road
Finchley
London
England
Great Britain
Europe
Northern Hemisphere
Earth
The Solar System
The Milky Way
The Universe

I think a lot of children do that as they emerge from the solipsism of early infancy. There is a stage where the only reality that matters is the one you can see. When you start to see beyond, there is a giddiness at the adjustment of scale. You play with the zoom on the lens to see how small you can make yourself in relation to the world, while still being its centre.

Over time, we lose that elasticity of perspective. Our sense of place hardens. The outer reaches fade from view. Somewhere along the line, our usual location is also imbued with a feeling of belonging. This is home, defined by the presence of family and feelings of security. It doesn't have to be a building. It is a space defined by familiarity. It is the place where nothing you say or do is alien to the people who call that same place home, because they know you as well as you know yourself, or better. 'Make yourself at home,' we say to someone when we want to indicate the opposite of being a stranger.

That is what makes the idea of a homeland powerful. It is the country where you cannot be an alien, even to people you don't know, because there is a common culture. Strangers are bound to each other by shared language, food, music, history, stories. In politics, the concept of a homeland is commonly bundled together with the idea of a nation, although in the long run of human social evolution, that is a recent development. The organization of cultural, religious and ethnic communities into distinctly national identities dates back to the eighteenth century. The aspiration to organize those groups into discrete countries with their own flags and anthems only picked up serious momentum in Europe in the nineteenth century. Usually, it grew from resistance to imperial rule or, for the empire-controlling nations, as part of the drive to consolidate imperial identity and repress those resistance movements.

Nationalists do not like to admit that the whole concept of a national homeland is that modern. For them, politics is the business of mobilizing people based on identities that have existed for millennia. Forever. That involves a lot of story-telling. History must be selectively narrated to cast a particular group – the nation – as the lead protagonist. We, the national tribe, must be the heroes. We overcome obstacles and vanquish enemies to fulfil the greatness for which we are destined – or look destined if events past and present are plotted on a particular line.

That line does not necessarily track historical reality. Mean-while, other nations are drawing their own lines on different trajectories, often using the same historical points. There are problems where the lines intersect. One nation's victorious battle of liberation is another's tragic loss of ancestral territory. One people's driving out an oppressive colonist is another's massacre by savages. That is how nationalism becomes such a powerful and self-sustaining engine of conflict. It is a perpetual grievance machine that excavates memories of enmity, steeps them in present resentments, refines them into fissile material and loads them up into political arguments.

Much of what looked like politics in the Baltic at the start of the twenty-first century was wrestling over control of twentieth-century history.

I had a lot of sympathy with countries that had been trampled by more powerful neighbours for generations. They were trying to reflate a culture that had been flattened by the Soviet monolith. That sympathy wore a bit thin when it came to Riga's annual celebration of the partisan legions – veteran soldiers who had resisted the Red Army on its way to Berlin in 1944. To most Latvians, the 'legionnaires' were national heroes fighting a desperate battle against Russian reoccupation. Awkwardly, those battalions had also been under the command of the Waffen SS. It took some effort of diplomacy by NATO and EU dignitaries to persuade the Latvian government that if they wanted to join the clubs of Western democracies they needed to drop the Nazis from their summer parades.

Growing up in Britain, I acquired what I thought was the standard version of the Second World War. The narrative has its beginning, middle and end, passing all the famous landmarks on the way. Germany invades Poland; Dunkirk; the Battle of Britain, etc. It builds to a crescendo for D-Day, and then victory. But there were other wars within the war. Other war *stories*. For Americans, it starts with Pearl Harbor and there is no Blitz. France venerates its resistance and glosses over its collaborators. All the Western Allies play down their reliance on the Soviet Union. The atomic annihilation of Hiroshima and Nagasaki is not much mentioned in victory commemorations. Some perspectives have been mythologized in multiple movie renditions. Others – the view from possessions of the British Empire, for example – not so much.

But the least familiar version, and the one I was not prepared for when I moved to the Baltic, was the story in which the Second World War lacks a happy ending. The Germans themselves conceded pretty quickly after the war that the Nazis losing it was a good outcome. Jews don't see any flex on that point.

But living in countries that lost their independence to the Red Army, I noticed ambivalence. It was mostly discreet, but it would sometimes spill into the open. Third Reich memorabilia of the kind that is illegal in Germany was sold at flea markets. In the years that I lived in Riga, I don't think I ever heard a Latvian say bluntly that the wrong side won the Second World War, but the national story contained a discernible lament about the way things had played out in 1945. For the Balts, the Second World War ended when independence was restored to their interwar republics. That was 1991.

The Holocaust is not the most memorialized atrocity in Baltic history. That place is taken by Stalin's deportation of Latvians, Lithuanians and Estonians to Siberia and other remote parts of the Soviet empire. The recapture of Baltic territories after the war was followed by indiscriminate punitive relocation of 'anti-Soviet elements'. Hundreds of thousands of men, women and children were shipped to the Gulag, put to forced labour or executed.

That trauma is seared into the collective memory. It evolved, as such traumas do, into a morality tale of national suffer-ing and redemption. Of course, that made idols of the freedom fighters who had resisted annihilation by Stalin's hand and kept the flame of nationhood alive. That some of those men were also eager Nazi collaborators was not a welcome caveat to the story.

I found that disturbing at first. I came to understand how it happened. Then to realize that it isn't unusual.

All national stories involve elisions to expunge crimes from the historical record. In Britain, there is no settled account of empire because it is so hard for people to admit that it was an enterprise fuelled by the economics of slavery, justified by doctrines of white racial supremacy. No nation wants to admit to itself that some of the people it has lionized as champions are also murderers.

Updating the national story so it aligns with historical truth is something democratic politics finds difficult. To understand why, it is necessary to take a step back and look at how democracy is supposed to work and what politics is for; what it is.

(iii) The inverse Clausewitz principle

Carl von Clausewitz, the Prussian general, defined war as 'a mere continuation of politics by other means'. Precisely what he meant by that is disputed by political and military theorists, as well as translators, who quibble over the emphasis implied by the original ('*Der Krieg ist eine bloße Fortsetzung der Politik mit anderen Mitteln*'). Setting those debates aside, I like Clausewitz's maxim more when it is inverted. In that form it becomes a statement about peace: politics is the resolution of conflict without recourse to war.

For most of history, when rival groups of people have failed to resolve their differences, they fight it out. The most effective mechanism ever invented for preventing that from happening is democracy. It awards different social and economic interest groups representation and an institutional framework for negotiating their differences. When it works, democracy makes violence redundant as a means for settling political scores. I call that the inverse Clausewitz principle.

It is easy to get used to the benefits conferred by that mechanism and then forget how they came about. That complacency breeds impatience with the operation of democracy. Democracy can be unwieldy and inefficient. It doles out disappointments as well as rewards. That is where populism seizes its opportunity.

The difference between populism and democracy is not

always easy to define, because all populists define themselves as democrats. They claim to be channelling a purer and more efficient kind of popular representation. They are wrong, and the reason is because populism violates the inverse Clausewitz principle.

Democracy is a mediation between rival interests. Finite budgets have to be allocated; taxes have to be raised from some people so the proceeds can be spent on others. One person's affordable housing scheme is an eyesore in another person's back yard. Democratic politics aspires to settle those questions in ways that leave more people satisfied over time than aggrieved. It also offers the aggrieved group a realistic expectation of redress down the line.

Everyone gets to feel represented, whether by government or opposition, which means we all buy into the continuity of the system. There are parties, campaign groups, trade unions, all channelling the various interests. They send politicians to parliaments, where deals are struck and compromises hammered out without anyone literally being hammered. The different factions test the popularity of their ideas (or, more commonly, the popularity of leaders advocating ideas) in elections. If the vote is free and fair – and perceived as such by the electors – everyone accepts the outcome.

The losers might not be happy, but they consent to be governed by the winners on the understanding that another vote will come around in due course. If the side that won last time has disgraced itself, they are punished. Losers' consent is a cornerstone of democracy. (It is why Donald Trump's refusal to concede the 2020 US presidential election to Joe Biden represented such a deadly assault on the constitution of the

American republic. It is also why Remainers misunderstood the offence caused by the suggestion of a second referendum after their defeat in 2016.)

There are courts to make sure the rules are not broken. There is an independent, free press to expose malfeasance and injustice. There is no need for revolution, in theory, because the ballot box is a pressure valve. It gives vent to forces that might otherwise demand that the ruling elite and its institutions be destroyed.

There is an unspoken social and economic contract under-writing these arrangements. Democratic politics makes civil war unnecessary, and in the absence of fighting, everyone is better off. We get to lead longer, more secure lives. With that interest in common, everyone is on the same side when it comes to the overarching principle of sustaining democracy itself. Partisan rivalries can be intense, but they don't bring down the system.

That is the theory.

There is a catch. In exchange for most people getting *some* of what they want *some* of the time, no one gets *exactly* what they want *all* of the time. And there will be points where decisions must be made for the long-term health of society that make a lot of people – perhaps even the majority – unhappy in the short term.

That is why elections are spaced out over cycles of four or five years. A government needs the chance to make some tough calls – raise taxes, cut spending, regulate activities that are fun but unhealthy – and if those calls turn out to have been the right ones, the initial anger dissipates. If every decision were subject to a referendum, that essential gap between a policy choice and its consequences would not exist. If there are no parties, and everything comes down to a beauty contest between charismatic leaders or a yes/no question, there is less scope for compromise once the votes are counted.

This is the difference between representative and direct modes of democracy. Representative democracy rejects as impractical and dangerous the idea of deciding policy by a vast national show of hands. Decisions are made in parliaments by politicians who exercise judgement on behalf of the people. MPs are expected to have the people's interests in mind, but not to give them instant gratification, which can't be done. Not for everyone at once.

As David Runciman, politics professor at Cambridge, has written:

> [Representative democracy] depends on the spaces that exist between the people and their politicians; between the taking of a decision and its evaluation by the public; between the act of will and the act of judgement. It depends on there being enough time to reflect on what we have done. It presupposes disappointment. It is a deeply frustrating business.

It is essential that citizens in the democracy tolerate that frustration; that they accept the imperfections of the system in recognition of its superiority to the alternatives. That frustration is also what gives populism its appeal and what defines it as distinct from democracy. A representative system demands patience and deferral of gratification from its citizens. Managing the various competing interests in a society is complex. Any problems that register as politically important will by definition be hard to solve.

Populism trades in bogus simplicity. It cultivates impatience and treats caution in the face of complexity as illegitimate dissent. The populist rejects the suggestion that problems are hard to solve as a lie told by an incumbent elite that is serving itself or making excuses for its failure to deliver free goodies for all. While democracy is the art of managing the variegated wills of different social groups, populism asserts that there is one unified and indivisible will of the people. The populist candidate is the embodiment of that will. His rivals, by extension, are enemies of the people.

But in rejecting the complexity of problems facing government, populism is destined to fail at the practical side of administration. It is then forced to govern in a state of perpetual campaigning aggression. A populist leader will end up having no choice but to use their power to silence or delegitimize critics. They need scapegoats to blame when their plans go awry. When they bungle economics, they steer the fight to culture.

A democrat asks to be judged by voters on achievements in office. A populist plays the victim even after a term in office. They recast themselves as martyrs for the people, denied the chance to achieve great things by sinister forces lurking in society, deep state subterfuge, foreigners, or a seditious media peddling fake news. The defeated populist never concedes.

Populists are sore losers but also sore winners, because the day after an election they face all the awkward, tricky problems of government that their campaigns have denied. They fail to deliver what they have promised and turn bitterly on the defeated parties who warned them it would be so.

Nationalism is a subset of populism. Both tend towards violation of the inverse Clausewitz rule. No government can meaningfully express the needs of a whole nation, united and indivisible. Nations house many incompatible wills that need mediation. A regime that denies that challenge will always end up in conflict with the principles of representative democracy. And, if unchecked, in other kinds of conflict.

Nationalists and populists always fail at practical policy. They cannot admit that failure, but it burns within them, lighting the hunt for traitors and saboteurs.

(iv) The concertina effect

The past should get more distant with age. Time passes, today becomes yesterday, shoving yesterday into the day before yesterday. The news gets old and then becomes history, which turns ancient. But it doesn't always feel like that. Not in politics.

There are periods when history is remote and moments when it rushes up to meet the present. The communist regimes of central and Eastern Europe had their own way of narrating the past to fit the template of Marxist theory. In that telling, nationalism was obsolete in countries that were governed by the higher principle of proletarian solidarity. In reality, nationalism was locked in ideological permafrost. When Soviet control melted away, old borders reappeared on the map; old grievances sprang back to life; old scores were suddenly unsettled; history that had seemed old barged into the present.

In the Baltic states, 1941 was a lot closer to 2001 than it had seemed to me in Britain. It felt as if history, instead of always receding into the past, could move up and down the timeline, folding towards the present like a concertina if the right political pressures were applied; if certain buttons were pushed, keys were played and an old half-remembered melody came out, triggering a rush of collective feeling.

The concertina effect is a function of political stress. A squeeze is applied and history groans and wheezes into life. Decades fold up into moments. I have felt it happening to Britain in recent years, starting probably with the Brexit referendum. The apparently simple proposition on the ballot paper – should Britain stay in the European Union or not – concealed a more profound challenge to national identity. It asked probing questions about what kind of country we were, what trajectory we were on and how that related to the place we had been in 1974, when Britain joined the European Community.

Those questions have never been absent from British politics and they weren't the explicit topic of most debates during the 2016 campaign. But Brexit closed the concertina. It gave the low hum of history a shrill salience. It armed stories about the past with emotional urgency and rammed them into the present.

The facts about Britain's relationship with Europe since 1974 have mostly been folded out of the picture. Banal realities of trade and diplomacy didn't make rousing melodies or stirring soundtracks to a culture war. The history that has ended up feeling suddenly closer to the present is not the chapter that was ostensibly contested in the referendum but older stories with a deeper purchase on national identity – the Second World War; the legacy of Empire.

Reckoning with history is a normal part of politics. Each generation has its turn at revising the record to accommodate changing values. But it is unhealthy for debate about bygone eras to subsume the politics of the present, as if the issues of today are mere shadows on the wall cast by flames of ancient grudge or glory.

That is a distortion of the concertina effect, making it impossible to consider the past without partisanship. It is felt in the strangely frenetic arguments that penetrate the news from time to time over who should be honoured with statues and whose monuments should be toppled, whether 'Rule, Britannia!' is a heroic anthem for all times or a vile celebration of colonial oppression, what the correct level of deference, if any, to a Union Jack should be and whether British schoolchildren should be taught reverence or atonement for the acts of their country's former rulers.

Brexit didn't start those fights, but it raised the temperature in ways that excluded cooler heads from the conversation. Much of the combustible material, especially on matters of race, has been imported from the US. The two countries' histories on that score are very different, but the political dynamics are aligned enough for ideological sparks to jump the gap. And once the fire has caught, there are many political incentives to fan the flames. There is an intensity to controversies around history and identity that is hard to resist for a campaigning candidate, especially one with a weak record in government to defend.

What defines the nation? Where did it come from? What does its flag represent? Those questions make a more intimate connection with audiences than the ones posed by dry disquisitions on budget allocations. But there is also a polarizing charge in that connection – a force of positive or negative association that pulls one tribe in close while repelling the opposite side.

It is possible to discuss history in a style that weighs evidence and considers context; that looks for the line of truth, notes how it diverges from the decorative lines that nations draw to celebrate themselves, and seeks calmly to explain the gap. But that is low-octane politics. It should be possible to recognize simultaneously that Winston Churchill's attachment to empire was steeped in racism and also that his war leadership was instrumental in saving civilization. The same flag that was flown in one time and place as a banner of justice and liberation might have been planted in a different place and time at the site of a massacre.

It is easier to accept those contradictions when the concertina is stretched wide; when the past feels old. When the history feels packed tight, the concertina has a higher pitch. There is a claustrophobia about politics in those closing folds. It is darker there and harder to keep things in perspective.

'The past is never dead,' wrote William Faulkner. 'It isn't even past.'

Brexit asked Britain to decide how European it was, which got me thinking about Linkuva – the town I had seen at the start of the twenty-first century and the one my grandparents had left a hundred years earlier and the in-between times being squeezed into now. Like everyone with an immigrant back-ground, I have often been asked where I am from. On giving the correct answer – London, England – I am met with the inevitable follow-up. Where are you from *originally*?

It isn't necessarily a racially charged question. Not for me. I don't wear overseas ancestry in my skin (although diligent anti-Semites have been known to pick out the Jewishness in my features pretty efficiently). It is the name that prompts curiosity.

There aren't many Behrs in Britain. The best guess as to its origin is Germanic, meaning something like peasant; simple person, one who dwells in a *bur* – a rudimentary cottage.

Where am I from *originally?* South Africa was a one-generation staging post. Before that there was Lithuania, but Jews and Lithuanians were separate categories of people at the start of the twentieth century. They had their own individual national stories. Lithuanians spoke Lithuanian and had distinctly Lithuanian-sounding names. They called their capital Vilnius. Jews called the same city Vilna, where they spoke Yiddish. They had names like Behr, Gilman, Rinkunsky.

The term that more accurately describes the heritage is Litvak – the sub-genre of Jewish identity that belongs (or belonged) to a large swathe of territory in north-eastern Europe. The Litvak zone encompassed modern-day Lithuania but also a swathe of land that includes parts of Latvia, Belarus, slivers of Russia and Ukraine, chunks of Poland, including the parts that were once East Prussia. Most of the national borders that partition that land were not there, or were in different places, when my forebears called it home. They are scars left by twentieth-century wars.

It never occurred to me to describe myself as Lithuanian when I lived by the Baltic. My Lithuanian friends would have thought it weird. I told them about my ancestral connection to their national homeland, but it wasn't something we ever discussed. It didn't bring us closer.

I must have mentioned the day trip I took to Linkuva, but I don't remember being asked what I had found there. I'm not sure I would have known what to answer. A disused cinema that smelled of piss and was once a synagogue. A cemetery.

I loitered by the graves until I felt awkward and went back into town. I found Danite, my helpful local guide. She wanted me to meet her neighbour, who had been interested to know that there was a stranger around asking about Jews. Mrs Gorbuzenie was 70 years old, a slight woman wearing a head-scarf and a simple cotton dress with a flower print. She had grown up in Pashvitinys and had a good school friend who was Jewish. There was a photograph, taken in the late 1930s, of a small group of girls with knee-length skirts, tidy plaited hair, sitting in neat rows. Mrs Gorbuzenie pointed to herself and to her friend, who she called only by surname, Schneiderite – a Lithuanianized version of the Jewish name Schneider.

When the Germans came, a local priest hid the girl and spirited her away somewhere. Mrs Gorbuzenie didn't know what had become of her until she got a letter after the war. They corresponded a few times but then lost touch again. It was all very vague. The dates, times and places were hazy. They hardly made a complete story, just a faint line connecting some dots in history, a line that had its origin in the same place as mine. That was something. I was comforted that someone wanted me to know that Linkuva's Jews had not all been murdered. The will to remember was buoyant. It was carried across generations on a sea of forgetting.

I finished my tea and got the bus back to Vilnius. I had the return ticket folded inside my British passport. I felt a rush of gratitude for both documents. I was glad to be getting out of Linkuva and gladder still to be doing it without fear. I held my passport tight, like the stub of a winning ticket in the bloody lottery of twentieth-century Europe.

CHAPTER 2

PROMISED LANDS

By the rivers of Babylon, there we sat down, yea, we wept, when
we remembered Zion.

Book of Psalms

(i) Writing on the wall

The carpet is a browner shade of orange, locating our scene
in the seventies. It covers most of the downstairs area of a
three-bedroom Edwardian semi-detached house in Finchley,
suburban north London, including the patch of living-room
floor on which I am sitting. On a black-and-white rented
television Margaret Thatcher is moving into 10 Downing Street,
which gives the scene a date stamp: Friday, 4 May 1979, a month
before my fifth birthday. It must be an evening bulletin, because
both of my parents are watching. I want to be interested too
but can't sustain the pretence, and go off to play elsewhere.

It is the first time I can recall being aware of the news,
meaning things that are happening to people I don't know but
that for some reason matter enough that I should care. Such
events are few in the imagination of a nearly-five-year-old.
Far more significant than the advent of Tory government would

be the arrival later that year of a Sony Trinitron TV – owned, not rented. The eighties dawned in colour.

Of our new prime minister, I knew only one thing: she snatched milk. This information was broadcast in graffiti on a fence that flanked a section of the walk we took to nursery. In tall white capital letters, someone had daubed the words: 'Thatcher: Milk Snatcher'. It was a reference to the Conservative leader's stint as Education Secretary in Ted Heath's government, when a free ration of milk had been withdrawn from the nation's schools.

I didn't know the background story, but I was impressed by the graffiti. I had dabbled in light defacement myself, scrawling abusive comments about my older brother in books and on walls at home. But the 'Thatcher: Milk Snatcher' slogan was vast. I had never been so close to words that were taller than me. Also, it rhymed.

This is where political engagement begins – at the boundary between the world you know at home and the one you see in the news. It is formed by the events that cross between the concentric circles of belonging, the ones I had once drawn as my childhood address. House, street, borough, city, country, etc. How was it relevant to our little family unit in Finchley that Thatcher snatched milk? Would she snatch it from me?

I learned that Thatcher was our local MP as well as the prime minister. I started to assemble a mental map of politics, to learn its compass points and identify local landmarks. Then I learned how to locate myself on the map, and which way to face.

A year or two after 'Milk Snatcher' had been erased, a pair of white swastikas appeared nearby, on red brick pillars supporting a Victorian viaduct at the end of our road.

The far right had enjoyed a political surge in the seventies, although support was already tapering off in the Thatcher years. The Tories offered some of the same pungent flavours of nationalism, seasoned with middle-class respectability. That went down well with voters who wanted a more orderly society, and whiter neighbours, but preferred not to be associated with actual fascism.*

I understood nothing of these trends, but I knew a swastika when I saw one. I don't remember not knowing. There must once have been a period when I was unaware that with just a few brushstrokes you could describe the ambition to exterminate people like me. But the knowledge, once acquired, is so severe that it hushes the preceding innocence out of recollection.

It was a fundamental part of what it meant to be Jewish. The cultural part of that curriculum was learned at home, but there were also classes every Sunday morning at a local synagogue. I learned to read Hebrew and was told about people who had been slaves in Egypt before escaping to the Promised Land. Monday to Friday I sat in an ordinary classroom and learned about people who had been conquered by a man called William, fought wars over roses and fended off a Spanish Armada. There wasn't much overlap between the two stories, but that wasn't a problem. No one was making me choose between them.

I was heartened when a counter-vandal covered the swastikas with white paint. They reappeared the following week, this time

---

* In her memoir, Thatcher describes her approach to immigration policy explicitly in those terms, emphasizing the need to 'articulate the sentiments of ordinary people' to close off political inroads for extremists. In 1978, when still in opposition, she told ITV's *World in Action* programme that she was 'rather afraid that this country might be rather swamped by people with a different culture'.

in red. My older brother and I played in woods that were flanked by the viaduct. I had thought the biggest danger there was nettles. I didn't like to think there might also be Nazis.

If there were, they can't have been many. Even a whole battalion of nocturnal skinheads in our woods would have been outnumbered by Jews during the day. Like most immigrants, my parents had chosen their destination country on the recommendation of people like them. Émigré trails are beaten smooth by word of mouth. That is how my great-grandparents had learned that South Africa was a good place to raise a family when Lithuania started to feel like a good place to leave. Herd security makes the transition to a new life less alienating. Being white and middle class was also a big help with integration.

England has an ancient tradition of anti-Semitism, with a catalogue of medieval massacres and persecutions. In 1290, Edward I expelled all Jews from the land (no one mentioned that when noble monarchs were the topic in history). But by the late twentieth century, the ancient hatred had decayed into a sly, winking kind of prejudice, made up mostly of arch comments about money (we were mean with it) and noses (ours were too big). I remember one incident at school where someone had glued a coin to a desk. Everyone who passed tried to pick it up, but not all efforts were met with braying jeers. Only some elicited the raucous response. I didn't get the joke until it was explained to me with great mirth. 'It's funny watching how people of a certain religious persuasion can't resist.'

It was the teacher who said that.

We were not spat on and sworn at in the streets of Finchley, as happened to friends from other immigrant backgrounds. Nor was I ever told to go back where I had come from.

Our ethnic camouflage concealed a slow-burn immigrant culture shock. I was into my late teens before I began to appreciate how drastic the decision had been for my parents to quit the country of their birth and start up in a different hemisphere. Their first impression, common to many new arrivals in Britain, was that the weather and the people were in league to be unwelcoming – a cold, damp front.

The newlywed couple made the journey by boat in 1970, sailing over the new year to arrive in 1971, the cruise doubling as their honeymoon. That meant departing from a Cape summer and landing in a North Atlantic winter. They arrived well qualified for work – he as a doctor; she as a social worker – but without resources. The early years in London, when my brother and I were born, were overdrawn and underheated. But white South Africans didn't emigrate for economic reasons. The whole society was organized for their comfort by repression of the black majority. Apartheid allowed the urban middle classes a lifestyle that their British counterparts could never afford – big houses, big gardens, maybe swimming pools, always servants. The cost in suppressing moral qualms was set by the individual conscience, and as history repeatedly shows, people award themselves a bargain at that price. Denial was an option, but ignorance of the injustice was not. To stay meant complicity. The other choices were resistance or flight.

Resistance was the heroic path, which is to say a dangerous one. To be active in the anti-apartheid movement invited attention from the vicious Bureau of State Security, known by the Orwellian acronym BOSS, masters of intimidation, torture and assassination. My parents dabbled in protest as university students, but you did not have to go far down that road, or even park your car on the road where the meeting was being held, without hearing footsteps behind you and having your licence plate number noted down.

The deeper into the struggle you got, the more hazardous it became. If the ambition was to raise a family free from denial and fear, there was only one option left – exile.

(ii) Inner emigration

Some émigrés wallow in reminiscence about the old country. They romanticize the life left behind and pay cultural tribute to it alongside their newly settled identities. Apartheid closed that channel to us. White South African nationhood was politically contaminated, not something to be embraced.

But a rounded sense of Britishness didn't spring up over-night to fill the void. Jewishness did that, even though we rarely went to a synagogue and observed few of the domestic rituals. We didn't keep a kosher kitchen and only ever mentioned God when taking His name in vain.

South Africa still had a magnetic pull on our attention. When it came to following the news, Soweto felt closer than Westminster. It often featured in the evening bulletins because of the increasingly vicious methods employed by the South African government to enforce apartheid and the unstoppable momentum of resistance. When scenes of rioting and burning townships came on the TV, the volume would go up and my brother and I would be hushed silent. No Tory minister was as familiar, nor as reviled in our household, as P. W. Botha, hard-line architect of South Africa's military state of emergency in the eighties.

My early-years orientation in British politics was made simpler by Mrs Thatcher's indulgence of Botha and her refusal to impose sanctions against his government. Such wickedness made the whole milk-snatching allegation all the more plausible.

I was aware of something different about our household that I could never name as a child. It didn't match the usual British idea of foreignness, which involved strange languages and exotic foods. We were un-British in a way that was private, invisible to the naked eye. It was the smattering of Hebrew, Yiddish and Afrikaans that my parents wove into their conversation if the topic was meant to be off limits to children. It was the fact that we called our mother Mom, and not Mum or Mummy like English children. As a family we were not demonstratively close to one another, but we had a code that knitted us tight. We had a way of looking at the world beyond our front door and of navigating the concentric circles of belonging that felt unique to us. It was the silent language of exile, described once by the American poet W. S. Merwin as 'freighted with richness no common tongue could offer'.

Part of that was a distortion of mental geography that gave proximity to distant lands and shrouded most of my own country in a fog of ignorance. We spoke all the time of Cape Town and Johannesburg, their landmarks, their distinctive accents. We very rarely left north London, having no relatives or old family friends to visit in other parts of the country. My brother and I were Londoners before we were English, and we were English most when we felt the need to defend the country of our birth against disparagement by our parents. They would mutter in frustration at how awful the place and its people could be. 'But *we're* English,' we would say.

Growing up as a second-generation immigrant is to live in a half-adapted state between belonging and pretending. It is like wearing the right uniform in the wrong size, or woven from an itchy fabric that you can tolerate in public but can't wait to remove when home. You are pulled between attachment to your private, secret family realm and the need to escape it. You are protective of the parents whose cultural separateness is the foundation of your own identity. But you also harbour resentment for the awkward shape of that identity – the way it doesn't slot neatly into the country you call home.

You feel you have had to work out for yourself how to be something that everyone else seems to be without effort. There is a feeling that your identity is an encryption to which very few people will get the key.

Then you grow older and get to know more people and learn about their families and childhoods and realize that the encrypted feeling is very common. You realize how many people are struggling to fit in; how movement between social classes can be as much a kind of exile as movement across continents. You learn that homelands are places inhabited and abandoned mostly in the imagination.

Exile is a state of mind that can be induced by all kinds of upheavals, traumas, family break-ups and breakdowns, alien-ations and disengagements. It doesn't have to be a function of migration. In the communist regimes of Eastern Europe, political dissidents would talk about 'inner emigration'. Denied the freedom to travel abroad, they would find sanctuary in a private recess of the mind. They would disengage from the external world of politics, inhabiting it only as a performance of themselves because that was what the regime demanded. Their real selves would be elsewhere, indoors, inside, shared only with the trusted few, or with no one.

Democratic politics should not induce that level of disengagement. If something about the tone, the style, the temperature of mainstream political culture provokes people into flights of inner emigration, it is a symptom of democracy malfunctioning.

(iii) The face of the Gorgon

South Africa wasn't the only topic that could engage my parents' attention in the evening news, forcing me and my brother into silence. Anything about Israel would have the same effect. It was not a country they ever called home, but it was a place that made a claim to be a homeland for people like us, whether we called it that or not. It was also the place we went on holiday every summer throughout my childhood.

In 1977, my grandparents on my father's side retired to Netanya, a Mediterranean resort around 30 kilometres north of Tel Aviv. The choice had been made on the basis of a provision in the will left by my great-grandfather.

Ber Levin had been a shopkeeper in Pashvitin, down the road from Linkuva. At some time around the turn of the twentieth century, he switched to being a shopkeeper in a village thousands of miles away, in the Karoo – South Africa's sprawling desert plain – where his shop was less likely to be destroyed in a pogrom. He was a devout man and a committed Zionist. He believed that Jews should aim to return to the Holy Land from which they had spent millennia in mournful separation. He hoped to facilitate a small part of that repatriation with the first clause of his will: 'It is my wish and desire that my children shall live in Palestine.'

Ber Levin's daughter Betty, the eldest of seven and my grandmother, was the only one who obeyed. She settled in a small two-bedroom flat with her husband, daughter and two grandchildren. My grandfather died in 1979 (a heart attack, of course) and my grandmother was hopelessly ill-equipped to navigate the administrative side of her emigration to a chaotic Middle Eastern country of which she had known practically nothing before departure. Every summer there was always a hideous ball of bureaucracy and financial neglect for my dad to disentangle. The stray ends would then form some new, even more convoluted knot by the following August.

It can't have been very relaxing for my parents. For me and my brother it meant mornings playing on the beach, punctuated by ice cream and bomb scares. Afternoons were a purgatory of bored incarceration behind closed shutters, electric fans on full, forbidden to venture out into the roasting heat.

The flat in Netanya came to feel a bit like home from home. If I examine that feeling more closely, or the memory of a feeling, I can also find relief from the duty of cultural adaptation that hung over our lives in Britain. That is another common part of the second-generation experience – having places in other countries that operate as embassies of your unassimilated identity; locations where you get to be your private self, the encrypted person you are with family. You can still feel foreign in such a place, but not alien.

Despite successive years travelling to the country, I stayed detached from Israeli society. I had learned to decipher the Hebrew alphabet and knew a bunch of impractical phrases from religious ceremonies, but I hardly picked up any of the modern language. Knowing how to thank the Lord for bringing forth fruit from the vine doesn't get you far when what you want is an ice lolly and you have to pay for it.

Israel was also a frantic country. The soundtrack to each morning was a chorus of car horns and indignant hollering. In a shop or café, waiting politely to be served meant forfeiting any prospect of service. The roads were lawless. Signs designating speed limits and one-way streets stood as poignant memorials to the unfulfilled intent of their municipal designers. Behind closed doors, people were warm and hospitable. On the street, at the bus station or in any official setting, the mood was sharp-elbowed, abrasive.

I understood little about Israeli politics. During the years we visited, the left-wing Labour Party that had dominated government since independence in 1948 lost its grip on power. The right-wing Likud party was in the ascendant, installing its first prime minister, Menachem Begin, in 1977. In 1979, Israel surrendered Sinai to Egypt in exchange for recognition and peace. In 1982, it occupied southern Lebanon. These events passed over my head, literally. We once went on a camping trip in Galilee, in the north of the country, and lay awake listening to the sound of rockets and small-arms fire crackling over the border.

The stories I heard from Israelis were one-sided: a morality tale of plucky self-defence against Arab aggressors who had wanted to suffocate the infant nation at birth. Of the plight of Palestinians, evicted, expropriated, driven from land in the process of Israel's foundation – *al Nakba*, the catastrophe, as it is known in Arabic – there was never any mention. It is one of modern history's cruellest tragedies that Jewish sanctuary became Palestinian exile. But that was never discussed, whether through ignorance, denial, fear or prejudice it is hard to say. There is no way to sift the ingredients of a silence.

There were guns everywhere, mostly slung over the shoulders of the young men and women, teenagers sometimes, fulfilling their obligatory national army service. Now that I have reached middle age, I see that those soldiers were still practically children.

There was a quivering tautness to the Israel of my childhood, as if the whole country were a temporary structure, a canopy pegged into the desert, the guy ropes clenched in the knotted fists of the generation that dreaded annihilation. Their memory contained one near miss already. The character of the country was marked by the violent trauma of its birth. Decades later, you could feel the defiant antagonism in the air, the panting breath of a people that had barely made it out of Europe alive.

Not everyone who completed the flight left the terror behind. There was a woman who sat on the low stone wall outside the apartment block that was our home for the summer holidays. I remember her as elderly, but she might have been younger than she looked. We knew only two things about her: that she lived in one of the apartments in the building and that she was a survivor.

There is no word that carries as much moral and historical freight in the vocabulary of Jews. Even as a child, when someone of that generation was described as a survivor, I didn't have to ask what she had survived. We knew enough to know how little we could ever know. It is such a potent term in the context of the Holocaust that I hesitated to use the same word in the title of this book. I worried that it might be misinterpreted, calling out from the shelf with a misappropriated credential – one that belongs only to those who went to that darkest of places and came out alive.

Mine was a mundane survival; this is my guide to engaging with politics that are incomparably benign when compared to the Third Reich. The only point of connection I dare to make is that growing up in the shadow of that horror, even at a remove of two generations, has a particular effect on the political imagination. It dissolves confidence in any informal social convention as a guardrail against evil. It facilitates the hypothetical extrapolation of nasty rhetoric into actual threat and ugly politics into worst-case scenarios. It is a bag always packed by the door, containing an answer to the question that arises in times of political crisis: 'How bad can it get?'

What had she seen, this silent spectre of a woman with the aura of detachment? She wore a grey woollen cardigan and a long, wide skirt, even in the fierce summer sun. She clutched a small black handbag and monitored the pavement hardly blinking. Sometimes she shuffled up and down the road.

Whoever she had been before the camps, or whichever part of the anti-humanity machine she had passed through, was not for us to know. She was not a frightening presence, although her fixed stare made us shy. A gentle smile sometimes rippled across her face, but there was a hollowness in her eyes; a depth that told you of a realm not anchored to our world. It was not a vacant look. It showed the reflection of some unfathomable void. It isn't a look you forget.

There is a line in Primo Levi's last and most guilt-stricken work, *The Drowned and the Saved*, published in 1986, a year before his death by suicide:

> We who survived the Camps are not true witnesses. This is
> an uncomfortable notion which I have gradually come to
> accept by reading what other survivors have written,
> including myself, when I re-read my writings after a lapse
> of years. We, the survivors, are not only a tiny but also
> an anomalous minority. We are those who, through
> prevarication, skill or luck, never touched bottom. Those
> who have, and who have seen the face of the Gorgon, did
> not return, or returned wordless.

It is not true, as the cliché has it, that history is written by the winners. But it is never written by the wordless.

The trauma for many who survived consisted not just of the depth of the abyss, but the fragility that was exposed in the civilization that fell into it. European culture and history, the legacy of the Enlightenment, the refinement of art and literature, every magnificent monument to humanity's power to improve itself – none of it had stood as a bulwark against evil. Or, as George Steiner put it, 'Goethe's garden almost borders on Buchenwald.'

In one of my first jobs, I had a colleague from Bosnia, a young Muslim woman whose family had found asylum in Britain when their country was torn apart by civil war. I don't know how we got on to the subject, but on one of our cigarette breaks the conversation turned to the relative ease with which law-abiding, peaceable citizens can be mobilized to participate in genocide, if the propaganda and incentives are right. She told me about the flight from her village when the Serb army moved in; how they had loaded up possessions on the back of a truck and driven off while their neighbours picked over anything that was left behind. 'You don't forget the faces of the people you see looting your kitchen when they had been drinking tea there with you three weeks before.'

It might not be rational to extrapolate every bout of turbulence into the worst imaginable scenario, but the darkest resonances can't be unheard when the sinister chords are struck. That is where Israel fits into the identity of many Jews who don't live there, even if it is hardly articulated in those terms. It is the destination on a ticket out of the worst-case scenario.

For thousands of years, 'Israel' and 'Zion' had featured in Hebrew liturgy as a symbolic aspiration loosely tethered to geographic reality. There is a narrative thread that begins as creation myth and moves through Biblical parable, legend, ancient history, all the way to the present: God's promise to Jacob of a land for his progeny; the Exodus, wandering the wilderness; founding kingdoms and losing them; building temples and seeing them destroyed; the scattering of people around the Mediterranean shore and beyond. The Greek word is *diaspora* – a dispersal. The Hebrew word is *galut* – exile.

The ambition of returning to Israel, one day singing the Lord's song in Jerusalem, was an incantation for centuries. It was not until the late nineteenth century, when Europe was experiencing an epidemic of national awakening, that it evolved into a political response to a question posed by centuries of scapegoating and persecution. If Poles belong in Poland, Irish in Ireland, Greeks in Greece, Serbs in Serbia, what is the proper land for Jews?

Zion was an obvious answer, and also the most far-fetched. As a bid for the engagement of Jewish intellectuals it faced ideological competition from socialism, which promised emancipation without relocation. A proletarian revolution would eliminate all suffering, thus obviating the need for oppressed minorities to found their own states. Meanwhile, to the most integrated communities in Europe's most sophisticated cities, the idea of a distinctly Jewish nation seemed irrelevant, or worse, a step back from modernity into superstition. For the well-heeled, bourgeois Jews of Vienna and Berlin, there was no need to go digging new homelands out of a desert in the Levant when they were every bit as Austrian and German as their Gentile neighbours. Those illusions were surrendered at the gates of Auschwitz. The survivors needed somewhere to call home.

(iv) Same difference

I was always relieved to return to London after holidays in Israel. My country was the one where it rained in August. I liked putting on long trousers, jumpers and socks again. That was a homecoming feeling. Still, the Mediterranean sun put a different complexion on things. I was not an Israeli by culture or citizenship, nor could I ever see myself becoming one. And yet Israel's national story was *about me* in a way that the one I was taught about Britain was not.

There had always been something arbitrary about my Britishness. I might just as easily have been American. My parents considered the US as the place for their fresh start before plumping for a destination where there was no risk of young medics being sent to war in Vietnam. Britain was home, but it lacked a folkloric purchase on the question of who I was, who my people were.

That didn't prevent me feeling attached to the place. I would define the bond as patriotic, although the ardour isn't unconditional, which some would set as the measure of true patriotism. Or is that nationalism? There is a lot of confusion about definitions. Sometimes nationalism is cast as a more aggressive version of patriotism; patriotism after a few pints of strong lager.

But the difference is more conceptual, and the different concepts are important. Patriotism is a feeling about the qualities of a country, identified in its culture and history. Nationalism is a political project that wants the state to define those qualities and wants government to police their expression. Patriotism is a celebration; nationalism is a mission. Both romanticize the past, but the nationalist pretends it can be reinstated as the future.

Patriotism can stay vague about the object of its veneration. You might feel patriotic about your country's music and sense of humour, while feeling embarrassed by its cuisine and ashamed of its record of colonizing other countries. It is spacious. The *patria*, the homeland, contains multitudes, and anything that happens there might be worthy of patriotism.

Nation is different. The word is used variously as a synonym for the land, the people who live there, their culture, and the state that governs them. In the mind of the nationalist it is all those things in one, but they don't always line up neatly together. In modern Western democracies lots of different cultures, ethnicities and histories jostle alongside one another untidily within the same borders. Under those circumstances, making a definitive list of features that describe the nation – a prescriptive menu of qualifying traits – is impossible. The attempt results in platitude and delusion. Forcing the issue tends towards violence.

The political scientist Benedict Anderson described nations as 'imagined communities', which is to say their existence – real enough in the minds of those who feel they belong in one – is a narrative construct. It is a myth that people tell themselves, assembled from bits of common economic interest, shared religion, ethnicity and remembered history. The myths stick and evolve into identities when they have sufficient resonance with a critical mass of people.

Those national myths are remarkably similar across countries, even when their function is to celebrate specialness. The pattern is almost universal. There have to be virtuous men (usually men) who secured the nation's territory with valiant exploits in battle. Often there are defeats too, which make the martyrdoms and grudges that differentiate one nation from its neighbours. There is a golden age, during which the people's natural talents blossomed under enlightened leadership. There is a dark time of captivity – or exile – when the nation was laid low, subjugated to the ways of foreigners or driven from its rightful terrain. The national flame came perilously close to extinction. Then there is the glorious liberation where it roars back to life.

One powerful galvanizing myth tells of the special deal that the nation has struck with God. The people are blessed by providence, bestowed with unique gifts that serve as a model to benighted foreigners and heathens. When Christian fund-amentalists from North America's bible belt to Northern

Ireland's Free Presbyterians want to depict themselves as heroic defenders of a besieged faith they reach for the Old Testament prophecy of Zion – the fable of God's chosen people and their Promised Land.

The theological underpinning of that manoeuvre is an argument that the Jews forfeited their claim to God's preference when they failed to recognize Jesus as their Messiah. That created a vacancy for a new chosen tribe who understood the Lord's message better than its original recipients.*

Not everyone with a strong sense of national identity is a nationalist, and not all nationalisms fit exactly the same mythological template. But they are remarkably alike, resembling each other most in the archetypal ways in which they insist that their qualities and stories are unique. I don't mean that as a denigration of nationalist sentiment. Visions of collective national emancipation have mobilized colonized and enslaved people to demand and seize their freedom. The principle that politics should be organized around the nation state was a vital stage in the evolution of secular democracy from the autocratic swamps of religious and aristocratic power in Europe in the eighteenth and nineteenth centuries.

It is after emancipation that the problems start, when the mobilizing energy of national mythologies must somehow be turned into a prescription for government; when the mythic power of collective nationhood collides with the practical

---

* This is one reason why fanatical Christian evangelicals identify so passionately (and politically) with modern-day Zionism. Another is paranoid fear of Islam blended with Messianic excitement at the idea of a Second Coming of Christ. Jews gathering in the Holy Land is a scriptural precondition for the fulfilment of Apocalyptic prophecy, so Middle Eastern conflict is all part of the plan.

reality of managing competing social and economic interests – the inverse Clausewitz principle. Then nationalism becomes a machine for manufacturing exile.

It is not a coincidence that the most extreme nationalist governments in history have ended up repressing minorities, banning political oppositions, starting wars and murdering people.*

There is also something desperate and absurd in the spectacle of politicians in mature twenty-first-century democracies and former imperial powers laying claim to the moral urgency of national liberation movements.

I remember speaking at a Brexit debate in 2016 where one of the pro-Leave panellists, a woman in her twenties, claimed that she had never lived in a free country, having been born in Britain when it was already under the colonial thumb of Brussels. An elderly Indian man in the audience challenged her. He had been born under the Raj. He had seen what colonial rule really looked like. He had witnessed families torn apart by the partition of India and Pakistan. The comparison with EU membership was grotesque, he said. Was she seriously trying to say that her experience was equivalent? Yes, she shot back, without hesitation. 'They are *exactly* the same.'

---

* That grim historical record is why so many contemporary nationalists are shy of the label. In August 2019, Nicola Sturgeon, who led a party that wears nationalism in its name, told an audience at the Edinburgh Fringe festival: 'I have some problems with that word because of the global connotations of it, but first and foremost I'm an internationalist.' Brexit nationalists have another mental obstacle to identifying themselves as such, which is the feature of English (national) chauvinism that supposes nationalism itself to be a continental mania and not something to which we, the pragmatists of Albion, are vulnerable.

(v) The socialism of fools

After I left home and went to university, Jewishness dropped out of my life. It wasn't forgotten, but nor did it occupy any prominence in my identity. And it didn't have any relevance to my engagement with politics, or none that was conscious and needed to be made explicit.

The man who changed that was Jeremy Corbyn. The Labour leader, chosen in 2015, had an unsavoury back catalogue of comradeship with apologists for terrorism against Israel and Jews, Holocaust deniers, anti-Semitic conspiracy theorists. He had invited them to the House of Commons. He also had a Praetorian Guard of digital defenders who viciously rounded on anyone on social media who flagged anti-Semitism as an issue.

I wasted enough time arguing with radical leftists online to grasp the logic of their position. Corbyn had been chosen as the paragon of socialist virtue. The measure of a true socialist was loyalty to him, and to criticize him was therefore to reject the principles of socialism. Jews were criticizing Corbyn. They were basing that criticism on 'anti-Semitism'. Ergo, the charge of anti-Semitism was itself something that only a non-socialist would level. It was being 'weaponized' against the Dear Leader because he criticized Israel; weaponized by right-wingers, Blairites, 'Zionists'. Corbyn could thus be declared innocent of anti-Semitism and his accusers declared guilty of an elaborate (Jewish) plot to smear him.

For voters who were not steeped in generations of factional left bickering, this whole controversy was baffling. But Corbynite anti-Semitism was a variant of the virus that had been circulating in the darker recesses of Marxist politics for decades.

There are two ways for anti-capitalists to arrive at anti-Semitism. The direct route links Jews with banking and exploitation of workers* – a deep well of cultural association, dug over centuries, tunnelling past medieval complaints about usury and reaching all the way down to Judas, pieces of silver and Pharisees.

Then there is the scenic route – via Israel. That argument goes as follows: capitalism, being always rapacious and exploitative, craves war and conquest. It is the engine of imperialism. Israel was carved out of Palestinian land, which had been a British imperial possession, and was colonized by white settlers from Europe (here, the theorist does not consider the refugee status of those arrivals and the question of where else they were supposed to go). Since Zionism is the doctrine that legitimizes the establishment of a Jewish homeland in Israel, it follows that Zionism is the apogee of imperialism, and racist. To be anti-Zionist is therefore to be anti-racist.

---

* This reasoning pre-dates the creation of modern Israel. Take, for example, J. A. Hobson, a radical economist and social scientist writing at the turn of the twentieth century. He was highly influential on the evolution of Marxist thought as regards imperialism, on which he wrote a seminal study in 1902. Central to his analysis is the role played by 'men of a single and peculiar race, who have behind them many centuries of financial experience'. These people 'are in a unique position to control the policy of nations'. Hobson goes on to clarify that wars of imperial aggression would not be possible 'if the house of Rothschild and its connections set their face against it'. In other writings, he was less euphemistic. In an account of the Boer War, he judged that the conflict had come about at the instigation and for the benefit of 'a small group of international financiers, chiefly German in origin and Jewish in race'. When his study on imperialism was reissued in 2011, the new edition included a foreword of lavish praise for the author's perspicacious and 'brilliant' analysis. That encomium was penned by Jeremy Corbyn.

Not all Jews are Zionists; not all Zionists are Jewish. It is possible to reject the political goals of Zionism (past and present) while not hating Jews. But it is hard to pull off that intellectual balancing act while denouncing Israel with flag-trampling, monomaniac fervour.*

Someone who despises a country as the epicentre of world villainy will struggle to prevent the animus spilling into their feelings about the people whose need for sanctuary that country was founded to meet. It is historically illiterate to suppose that self-certification in left-wing anti-racism is sufficient qualification to police that line.

It is also disingenuous to claim, as Corbyn's defenders still do, that anti-Zionism is misrepresented as anti-Semitism as a tactic to silence criticism of Israel. (Israelis manage to criticize their own governments all the time without going the extra step and volunteering to dissolve their country and throw themselves into the Mediterranean.) The cause of justice for the exiled Palestinian people is not well served by the Western leftists who conflate the state that oppresses them, via a mythologized global 'Zionist lobby', with all of world Jewry.

But 'Zionism' on the left is code. It allows people to despise a foreign country, to assert that its foundation was a crime and to endorse calls for its violent abolition while denying that there is any prejudice behind that rage. Anti-Zionism is an ideological conveyor belt that carries the most zealous opponents of

---

* It is harder still to maintain the distinction when the target is not a government and its policies, but a nebula of influence that is said to sustain Israeli wickedness – the ubiquitous and omnipotent Zionist lobby. Such broad-brush loathing engenders hostility to a lot of people who aren't Israeli citizens but do happen to be Jewish.

modern Israel towards older paranoias about shadowy Jewish networks of economic and political influence. There is a reason why German social democrats in the late nineteenth century referred to anti-Semitism as *der Sozialismus der dummen Kerle* – the socialism of fools.

I and my Jewish friends, all former Labour voters, saw the evidence pile up against Corbyn and wondered how egregious an offence would have to be to cool the ardour of his fans. The left, normally quick to denounce even the lightest brush with racial insensitivity, lavished the benefit of the doubt on its leader, as if by some extraordinary coincidence he just happened to keep turning up in the same room as anti-Semites; just happened to find himself standing in a sewer and never once remarked on the smell.

'I understand why Corbyn might offend you,' a pro-Labour journalist told a Jewish colleague in one of the many arguments we all had on this issue. 'But what exactly are you frightened of? I mean, there are not going to be pogroms.'

The last rampage on British soil deserving of that label was in the summer of 1947. The trigger was a story of terrorism committed by Zionist paramilitaries, impatient with Britain reneging on a pre-war commitment to establish a Jewish state in Palestine. Two army sergeants, Mervyn Paice and Clifford Martin, were kidnapped and murdered. Their bodies were hung up in an olive grove near Netanya. There was outrage back in Britain. Vengeance was exacted on shops and synagogues across the country: Glasgow, Liverpool, Hull and Plymouth. In Birmingham, a slogan was daubed across two blocks with the words: 'Gentiles Arise. Resist Jewish enterprise. Remember Paice and Martin.' In Eccles, Greater Manchester, a former sergeant major was arrested for addressing a crowd with the words: 'Hitler was right. Exterminate every Jew. Every man, woman and child.'

Even in twenty-first-century Britain, safe by any historical measure, the hearts of the survivors' grandchildren beat with a trace of inherited dread. It is the cautionary tale about the worst-case scenario that was handed down; it is the emotional baggage and the passport kept ready for sudden flight. It is the inescapable suspicion that no matter how rooted Jews feel in a country and its culture, one day there will come a mob armed with the rusty old prejudice to let us know that we don't belong.

As one Jewish friend said to me in Labour's darkest days, 'At least we are finding out who would have hidden us in their attic.' We laughed, because it wasn't even a joke.

CHAPTER 3

FINEST HOURS

What is a country? . . . A vast land and a table. It is a table surrounded by loved ones to whom you don't have to explain your jokes, and the vast land that surrounds it, which is mostly your imagination.

Ece Temelkuran

(i) Cool Britannia

I am looking at an old photograph, taken at a party that I think happened on New Year's Eve 1996 or maybe 1997. I can't be sure. My shirt is unbuttoned, and for reasons that the camera could not record, two flexible plastic baubles of the kind that disperse laundry liquid in a washing machine are attached to my chest, held in place by the vacuum created when the air is expelled. They make a pair of clown's red noses, but green, and nipples. My hair is worn in a floppy fringe of brown ringlets. I look slim, not unhealthy, with an idiotic grin. I am probably stoned. I am holding a big glass tumbler that contains what I suspect to be white wine. I am young, unattached (except to the laundry baubles), irresponsible, looking preposterous and happy. I have a job in London at the end of the Millennium. There might have been better times in history to be twenty-something

73

with money in your pocket. There might have been better cities, too. But I wasn't complaining about the hand I had been dealt.

The economy was on an upswing after a savage recession at the start of the decade. London was buzzing with cultural optimism, creative energy and, at the weekends, Ecstasy. In 1996, *Newsweek* magazine ran 'Cool Britannia' as its cover story, but we didn't need a steer from the Americans to know that we were already in the best capital city on the globe.

We didn't know that our local confidence went with a historical tide of complacency. It was an age when the good news seemed to outrun the bad. Nelson Mandela was free. There was a peace process in the Middle East. The one in Northern Ireland was working.

The Cold War had ended without the nuclear cataclysm that seemed plausible for decades. Eastern Europe's captive nations were free. Western governments had money to spare because there was less need to spend on defence. Businesses were expanding into markets that had been walled off from capitalism. The internet was new and exciting. In economics, the period has been described as the Great Moderation – a phase of exceptionally low volatility. For those of us who experienced it as our formative years, it was a duplicitous normal. We set our expectations of political stability and economic growth to a level that subsequent events have proved absurdly optimistic. It was our golden age, which is to say we were laying the foundations for a vast edifice of nostalgia.

What I have more recently found intolerable about British politics can only be properly diagnosed with reference to that glorious *fin de siècle*. To know the present feeling of exile means revisiting the country as it was when I felt most at home in it.

I graduated into Cool Britannia. I didn't even have monstrous debts, just a small overdraft. University tuition fees had been paid by the taxpayer. I signed up with an employment agency and told them I was not fussy about jobs. I stuffed envelopes, entered numbers into a spreadsheet, delivered mail around office buildings. I had a stint unpicking rusty staples from mouldy clumps of paper and feeding the pages into a shredder. I enjoyed it, because it put money in my pocket. Then I landed what felt like my first proper job, adjacent to something I thought I might want to do for a living. It involved scouring the press for reports of upcoming events and entering the details into a database. I wasn't writing in newspapers yet, but I was being paid to read them, which meant I was officially employed in the media. It was not lucrative. But you didn't need lucre in those days to rent a room in a shared house in a fairly central corner of south London.

Documentary evidence of what I got up to after work hours is mercifully scant. The laundry bauble photo is a rarity. We didn't have cameras in our pockets all the time. Mobile phones were still a novelty, not a compulsion, and not smart. We had all the technology we needed to arrange spontaneous mischief but not to capture it for posterity or share it in real time. It is one of the less acknowledged privileges of my generation: we got the thrill of being connected without the tyranny of being always on.

There is a quote usually attributed to Napoleon but not reliably sourced to him: 'To understand the man you have to know what was happening in the world when he was twenty.' In truth, you need a lot more information than that, but the tail end of adolescence is uniquely formative. We think we have grown up, but we aren't grown-up enough yet to feel the status as a burden. Maybe a worldview does get baked in by those conditions. Maybe it is also a feature of what the American journalist Joan Didion once characterized as 'one of the mixed blessings' of life in one's early twenties: '[T]he conviction that nothing like this, all evidence to the contrary notwithstanding, has ever happened to anyone before.'

The word nostalgia is derived from the Greek *nostos*, meaning a return – with the inference of a fond destination, a homecoming, like Odysseus's voyage back from the Trojan War to the wife he left behind.

Algos is pain.

The term nostalgia, painful longing to return, was coined in 1688 by Johannes Hofer, a Swiss doctor who used it as a diagnosis of chronic homesickness experienced by mercenary soldiers encamped far from their native country, who exhibited depressive symptoms of lethargy and unshakeable melancholy. So vulnerable was the Swiss army to this condition that the playing of a traditional milking song, 'Khue-Reyen', was banned – punishable by death – because it induced paroxysms of wistfulness.

Nostalgia continued to be seen as a disease through to the nineteenth century, and then, as modern psychology caught on, a mental disorder of some kind. Only relatively recently has it shed the pathological stigma. Today, some psychologists take a more generous view, seeing it as one of the mind's defences against trauma and alienation. The happy past, or rather, a happier idea of the past, offers a place of sanctuary from an otherwise inescapable present. In that interpretation, nostalgia functions as a vault of cherished positive memory – a resource of good vibes that we dip into to buy an emotional passage out of present discomfort. As the sociologist Fred Davis has written:

> [Nostalgia] reassures us of past happiness and accomplishment; and, since these still remain on deposit, as it were, in the bank of our memory, it simultaneously bestows upon us a certain worth, irrespective of how present circumstances may seem to question or obscure this. And current worth, as our friendly bank loan officer assures us, is titled to at least some claim on the future as well.

Why else would I feel fondly now about the hours I spent unstapling bundles of paper? Those were not the best times, but I remember them as a good time. It was a good time to *be me*. What did that guy have that I miss? Knees that don't twinge when you stand up suddenly? Arteries unclogged by cholesterol? Yes, those things. But something else, too – politics that went with the grain of my own preferences; a homeland.

That Greek root *algos* is visible also in *analgesia* – treatment for pain. Nostalgia, used as analgesic, is addictive. In excess, it is poison. Populists and nationalists mobilize nostalgia as a weapon to obliterate the complexities that make governing hard. Present woes, they say, exist because the better country you remember has been stolen. It can be recovered.

The late Russian-American theorist Svetlana Boym distinguished between two modes of nostalgia. There is the 'reflective' kind, which is wistful and also self-aware. It knows it is being nostalgic. Then there is the 'restorative' kind, which makes an ideology of the *nostos* – the homecoming. Restorative nostalgia doesn't think of itself as nostalgic or even subjective. It claims to be dealing in immortal truths and untouchable traditions that must be preserved or rehabilitated.

I know I can't get my twenties back. But the harder truth to take on board is that the politics of that time are also irretrievable. I might reflect on them fondly, mournfully. But to dream of restoration is a fallacy no less wrong-headed than the nationalists' habit of painting the future in mythic colours of the past.

(ii) Things could only get better

I was too young to vote in the general election of April 1992. Just. John Major comfortably beat Neil Kinnock (and opinion-poll forecasts) after 12 years of Conservative incumbency and two months before my eighteenth birthday.

When the next opportunity came, I had five years of pent-up suffrage waiting to be directed against the Tories. Meanwhile, the political wind had changed. On 16 September 1992 – Black Wednesday – the UK crashed out of the European Exchange Rate Mechanism. The Tories' reputation for sound economic management was ruined and the Major government descended into a bog of sleaze and infighting over Europe. The pendulum of public opinion, which had seemed for so long stuck on the right, broke free, loosened by Tony Blair's compromises with Conservative opinion and lubricated by his smile. It hurtled towards New Labour.

In 1996, Helen Fielding's fictional diarist Bridget Jones spoke for the nation (or at least that part of the national majority in which I felt comfily at home):

It is perfectly obvious that Labour stands for sharing, kindness, gays, single mothers and Nelson Mandela as opposed to braying bossy men having affairs with everyone shag shag shag left right and centre and going to the Ritz in Paris then telling all the presenters off on the *Today* programme.

On polling day, Thursday, 1 May 1997, even the weather seemed to agree that it was time for a change. The sun rose on one of those crisp spring days that cannot fail to light optimism in British hearts, trained by experience never to expect comfort from the weather. I stayed up all night cheering as a succession of stunned Tories were flushed out of what they had thought were safe parliamentary bolt-holes. The emblematic moment was Defence Secretary Michael Portillo's defeat in Enfield Southgate. *Were You Still Up for Portillo?* asked the title of a book narrating the drama of the night. Yes, was the answer. But I had cheered loudest when Finchley turned red.

'A new dawn has broken, has it not?' Tony Blair asked the crowd at a victory rally at the Royal Festival Hall. His theme song was 'Things Can Only Get Better' by D:Ream, a restless anthem of disposable pop exuberance. Its power to move me was out of all proportion to its limited musical merits, and survived subsequent political disappointments.

An electoral landslide buries subtle contours in the land-scape of national opinion.* Blair won 418 seats, giving him a Commons majority of 179. But his 13.5 million vote tally was

---

* This is especially true with Britain's first-past-the-post voting system, under which a landslide causes clods of electoral soil to heap up in ways that poorly represent the distribution of votes across the country.

less than the 14.1 million who had backed the Tories five years earlier.

Major's downfall was hardly the storming of the Winter Palace, but it had some of the character of a cultural revolution: a moment, like the Brexit referendum 19 years later, when the democratic process seemed to express a metamorphosis in national identity. In his election manifesto Blair had written that New Labour was 'the political arm of none other than the British people as a whole'. It was a silly assertion, and any leader making it now would be accused by liberals and the left of shabby populism. But at the time it was a plausible banality because there was such a settled consensus around the idea that the Tories' time was up, and Labour were the automatic alternative.

Blair's easy charm achieved something vital for success in a country that thinks of politics, like religion, as something better not discussed in social situations. He made Labour feel like the default setting, a place to be politically neutral.

It was a different style of dominance to the one Thatcher achieved after 1979. Blair swam the prevailing tide brilliantly. Thatcher built dams. She made it her business to re-engineer national consciousness. In 1981, she told the *Sunday Times*: 'Economics are the method: the object is to change the heart and soul.'

New Labour also moulded hearts and souls, but by stealth. In domestic policy,* the government was squarely in the social democratic tradition. It raised taxes and spent the revenue on

---

* Foreign policy is another story, confined to a footnote here not to belittle its significance but because it only became a defining feature of the New Labour legacy after 11 September 2001.

public services. But the leadership, scarred by successive election defeats, felt the need to smuggle that process past voters. The electorate's rejection of Kinnock's 1992 manifesto, hardly a blueprint for radical socialism but not shy about tax rises, taught a Labour generation to think that egalitarianism could only be brought to Britain furtively.

The architects of New Labour also understood that winning power in Britain involved a battle for control of national identity. More precisely, they understood that Tory implosion created an opportunity to address another chronic electoral vulnerability – suspicion that the left has a problem with patriotism. The resulting iconography was not subtle: an election poster featuring a British bulldog; a TV broadcast where 'Land of Hope and Glory' played over scenes of overcrowded hospitals as bitter comment on Conservative underfunding of public services.

Peter Mandelson called it reclaiming the flag. 'It is restored as an emblem of national pride and diversity,' he said. 'Restored from years as a symbol of division and intolerance.' In 1995, Blair declared that Labour was 'the patriotic party because it is the people's party'.

The left was (and still is) uncomfortable with that repositioning exercise. Tony Benn, long-serving prophet of aristo-puritan socialism, said Blair's deployment of the flag 'called to mind the National Front'.

Socialist squeamishness about symbols of nationhood is perennial. Each generation of activists has to relearn the same two lessons the hard way. First, most voters think of patriotism as a virtue and don't want to be made to feel like hooligans and bigots for venerating their flag. Second, it is better to find positive stories to tell about an inclusive, tolerant mode of patriotism than to cede the whole topic to people who will gladly project patriotic fervour through an angry divisive lens.

George Orwell, in *The Lion and the Unicorn*, wrote:

> England is perhaps the only great country whose intellectuals are ashamed of their own nationality. In left-wing circles it is always felt that there is something slightly disgraceful in being an Englishman and that it is a duty to snigger at every English institution, from horse racing to suet puddings. It is a strange fact, but it is unquestionably true that almost any English intellectual would feel more ashamed of standing to attention during 'God Save the King' than of stealing from a poor box.

That was written when the Luftwaffe were bombing London. Then consider the same point made 55 years later by another astute observer of the places where culture, politics and identity merge. In the run-up to the anniversary of the Nazis' defeat, Bridget Jones wrote in her diary:

> Is it possible to have a kitsch ironic VE Day party – like for the Royal Wedding? . . . No. You can't be ironic about dead people. And there's the problem of flags. Half of Tom's friends used to be in the Anti-Nazi League and would think the presence of Union Jacks meant we were expecting skinheads.

The same argument comes round whenever an anniversary or royal jubilee brings vast amounts of bunting into the street. There is reliably a confected and self-righteous row between polemicists and provocateurs of left and right over whether the spectacle is a portrait of national self-confidence or a sinister tableau of incipient fascism.

The iconography of Cool Britannia seemed to provide a respite from that tedious controversy. It was not a replacement for conventional pomp, but a rock 'n' roll rebrand. It was Britpop patriotism, saluting the Union Jack as an emblem of younger, metropolitan swagger. Bombast with irony. It was an illusion. But it allowed us to participate in the celebration of nationhood while reassuring ourselves that we were not endorsing the same things as the skinheads who happened to be parading the same colours.

The memo about moving on from deranged jingoism did not reach Fleet Street. When England faced Germany in a semi-final of the 1996 European football championships, the *Daily Mirror* famously ran a front page with Paul Gascoigne and Stuart Pearce mocked up in military helmets, under the headline 'Achtung! Surrender' (subhead: 'For you Fritz, ze Euro 96 Championship is over').

Germany won on penalties. That night, rioting England fans took out their frustration on police and street furniture in Trafalgar Square. The old marauding instinct had not subsided. In Brighton, a Russian student was mistaken for a German and stabbed.

The *Mirror*'s defence was that its front page should not be taken seriously, which was half true. It was not meant to be taken literally. But it was not a joke at England's expense. The depiction of Germany as the perpetual enemy spoke to a deeper emotional current in the national psyche that was not funny.

There is a tendency for liberals of my generation to

romanticize the late nineties* and early noughties as a time of radiant enlightenment when before had been Tory dark ages. Britain at the end of the New Labour era was less uptight and more tolerant than it had been at the start. In areas of sexual and racial equality the change was hastened by progressive legal reforms, although the balance of cause and effect is debatable. Blair was a shrewd reader of shifts in the national mood, which he played back to people as policy. A wider audit of Blairism (for which there is not space here) would reveal both liberal and authoritarian strands – enough to support divergent interpretations of the legacy† and material to sustain eternal rancour between left and right factions in Labour.

Looking back, it was no revolution if the measure is dismantling of conventional hierarchies of economic and cultural power. The upper echelons were still very white; mostly male. Trends that were discussed in all seriousness as progress in male emotional maturity and feminism – the 'new lads' and 'ladettes' – look flimsy in hindsight, little more than pretexts to move pornography from the top to the middle shelf.

The past always embarrasses itself in tests of virtue set by the present. But there is one scale on which the New Labour years register as a time of hugely significant cultural and political change, and that is the force of the political backlash when its moment came.

Shock at that reaction was also a measure of my complacency.

---

* A YouGov survey in 2019 that asked people to rank how favourably or unfavourably they viewed every decade since the fifties, regardless of whether they had been alive at the time, showed the nineties winning out over the rest.

† New Labour's record is especially messy when it comes to the subject of immigration policy – a problem to be met in Chapter 4.

I knew that fashions changed, but I really thought that the worst of uncool Britannia had been consigned to the dustbin of history. And for most of the New Labour years, the Tories worked hard to prove that judgement right. They inculcated a smug self-satisfaction in their enemies for which a terrible vengeance would be exacted.

(iii) Fruitcakes, loonies and closet racists

Democracy is easy to like when you are winning. Yielding to the justice of majority rule is painful when you are the minority. But hardest of all is admitting that your side deserved to lose.

This was not a problem I had to contend with between 1997 and 2010. I basked in the Tories' discomfort, bafflement and denial as Britain set sail into the twenty-first century, leaving its former party of power marooned on the shore.

It was Theresa May, then party chair, who in 2002 confronted a Tory conference with the character of its problem, which was a problem with its character. 'You know what some people call us – the nasty party,' she said. 'Our base is too narrow and so, occasionally, are our sympathies . . . The truth is that as our country has become more diverse, our party has remained the same.'

It took another election defeat, the third in a row, for that message to sink in. Then David Cameron embarked on the project that he called modernization and his supporters referred to as brand decontamination.

The exercise was not purely cosmetic, but nor did it go deep.

Cameron regretted none of Thatcher's economic policies but insisted that Tories make peace with the social changes that had accompanied New Labour. He exorcized a few of the uglier policy ghosts from the 1980s, conceding that opposing sanctions against apartheid and legislating against the 'promotion of homosexuality' had been wrong. There was a trip to the Arctic for a photo shoot with huskies to demonstrate his credentials as an environmentalist. There was a speech arguing that delinquent youth would benefit if everyone could 'show a lot more love'.

But in terms of what defined the Tories as a marginal sect instead of a national movement, the most significant of Cameron's instructions was the one to 'stop banging on about Europe'.

In the post-Brexit world, it is often forgotten that leaving the EU was a crackpot notion so recently. It was not the explicit demand of Tory Eurosceptics during the party's civil war over the Maastricht Treaty during John Major's stumbling retreat from power. In the 1997 general election, radical anti-Brussels sentiment was channelled by Sir Jimmy Goldsmith's Referendum Party, which demanded a plebiscite on EU membership. It got less than 3 per cent of the vote.

Europe was sometimes pertinent in British politics but rarely dominant for long. Britain's candidacy to join the single currency was a big issue in Blair's first term. His final years included a kerfuffle over ratification* of the Lisbon Treaty. EU enlargement to include former Warsaw Pact countries generated tabloid hysteria in expectation of a surge of Polish plumbers across the border. But quitting the Union was not proposed as a remedy in the political mainstream.

---

* Technically, Blair had promised a plebiscite on a different thing – an EU constitution that was obstructed by votes in other member states and was hastily refashioned into the Lisbon Treaty. The difference was subtle and, like so many European matters at the time, unremarked by the vast majority of people.

There was an asymmetry of interest and emotional investment. The people who liked the EU did so passively, vaguely and, for the most part, not knowing what it was they liked about it. They knew only that it was a weird fixation for the party that had disqualified itself from power.

Europe didn't register as something worth caring strongly about either way. Crusading against Brussels regulation was an alien preoccupation for the Cool Britannia crowd. London fashions were being displayed in Paris and Milan; British cafés embraced French pastries and Italian-style espresso-based coffees. Britain, newly at ease with itself as the capital of hip, found it easier to be relaxed with the rest of the continent. That left the sceptics caricatured as claret-faced Little Englanders, egg stains on their regimental ties, expectorating angrily about the forgotten merits of capital punishment.

For most of the New Labour years, liberal and left opinion measured Euroscepticism as a symptom of the wider reactionary syndrome that kept the Tories safely away from public affection. Cameron's modernization made his party competitive again, but the very fact that he saw monomaniac rage against Brussels as an impediment to that process confirmed that 'banging on about Europe' was electoral halitosis.

The prospect of that faction producing a governing majority was laughably remote. When Tory members elected Iain Duncan Smith as their leader in 2001, the choice seemed to confirm that the party was marching in the wrong direction.* He had been one of the Maastricht rebels whose parliamentary

---

* IDS has been completely rehabilitated since then, proving that political consensus can shift dramatically. In terms of what was good for Britain, the consensus can still have been right the first time.

guerrilla antics harried the Major government to its electoral grave.

The UK Independence Party was in its infancy then and a long way from causing any measurable political disruption. In the 2005 general election, UKIP took 2.2 per cent of the vote. Nigel Farage became the party leader the following year. Cameron was then still sufficiently confident that UKIP could be confined to the fringe that he described it as a collection of 'fruitcakes and loonies and closet racists, mostly'.

Nine years later, Cameron acquiesced to UKIP's central demand for a referendum on EU membership. He didn't doubt that the case for staying in would prevail, because he was a product of the era that heard a crackpot ring to the case for leaving and thought Britain was too sensible to vote en masse for cracked pots.

The huge imbalance of engagement on the European question is important for understanding how Brexit happened and why it discharged so much lingering poison into British politics. For years, the sceptics were passionate, deadly serious and deeply unfashionable. The pro-Europeans didn't even realize the fight had started. They correctly saw that voters didn't care about the EU and incorrectly thought that was what Euroscepticism was all about. They didn't see the seeds of a nationalist backlash against cosmopolitan liberalism and globalization. Why would they? The economic and political climate was still defined by the Great Moderation. The complacent tide was still rising.

(iv) Chucking rocks over the wall

One person who understood the mythic potency of Europe in the English imagination – and how to harness that power to personal ambition – was Boris Johnson.

When first appointed Brussels correspondent for the *Daily Telegraph** in the early nineties, Johnson found the task of serious reporting on European affairs boring. It was turgid technocratic stuff that he deemed unworthy of his destiny as a man of historical consequence. In response, he invented a new journalistic idiom, describing banal EU regulations in grotesque cartoonish terms. He inflated and distorted them to look like absurd plots by a malevolent bureaucracy: banning prawn cocktail flavour crisps; straightening bananas; limiting condom sizes to fit (presumably continental) small penises.

In an interview in 2005, Johnson described his technique as merry vandalism:

> Chucking rocks over the garden wall . . . I listened to this
> amazing crash from the greenhouse next door over in
> England as everything I wrote from Brussels was having this
> amazing, explosive effect on the Tory party – and it really
> gave me this, I suppose, rather weird sense of power.

---

*   Mostly, I don't think it is useful to depict newspapers as manufacturers of prejudice. They generally amplify existing trends. That isn't to claim any nobility on behalf of my trade, but simply to caution against a lazy analysis, common on the liberal left, that locates the roots of every defeat in media manipulation of a bovine public. That said, when it comes to informing the public about what the EU actually is and does, the British media has disgraced itself collectively, but that is for another chapter.

He was developing the gift that would later change the direction and character of British public life: the ability to mobilize powerful emotions with a message encased in levity, thus protecting the messenger from responsibility for his words; serious demagoguery dressed as a bit of mischief. 'Trolling' is the word now used for that vindictive mode of political provocation that tries to evade accountability by rejecting seriousness.

Johnson's method was so effective because it chimed with an older neurosis about Britain's relationship with its neighbours. It animated the oscillating complex that flips between superiority and inferiority – aloofness from peculiar continental manners and fear that those manners are somehow more sophisticated than ours. That tension has existed for hundreds of years. But it became particularly potent in the conservative imagination in the years after the Second World War, as pride in victory turned to confusion at the loss of imperial supremacy.

Britain joined the European Economic Community in a moment of strategic self-doubt and economic underachievement. By 1973, West German industry, flattened in 1945, had been rebuilt with Marshall Plan money to a higher spec than British rivals could manage. The recognition that modernization and prosperity required integration with the former foe when the ashes were still warm by historical standards was reached reluctantly; bitterly. Ungrateful France did not repay its liberators with humility. General de Gaulle had vetoed British EEC entry a decade earlier. The doors to the continental club were opened not on demand but after supplication.

Thatcher had been a supporter of entry, but with a certain grinding of teeth that was succinctly expressed in a TV interview in 1979, when the Tories were still in opposition: 'I can't bear Britain in decline, I just can't bear it. We who either defeated or rescued half Europe, who kept half Europe free when otherwise it would be in chains . . . and look at us now.'

Embarrassment is not often enough recognized as an engine of history, maybe because it is embarrassing to admit it as an individual motive. Most of our worst memories, the ones we wish we could delete from the mental record, are humiliations or acts of stupidity that can still induce a cringe decades later. Pain, the more dreaded sensation, is easier to bear over time. In memory it is vague and hard to summon. We adapt to loss. Wounds heal. Grief goes numb. A blocked artery can be propped open with a stent. But shame? Shame has a lingering burn. It commits relentless violence against the ego.

In the British nationalist imagination, a seed of shame was sown at the moment of entry into the European project because it was the inverse of what was commonly held to be our finest hour thirty years earlier. In military terms, victory over fascism was achieved by alliance with the Americans and the Soviets. But in cultural terms it was born of solitary defiance on an island fortress. It was the culmination of Churchillian resolve to fight on the beaches; the lone bastion of freedom in Europe. That episode filled British identity with vast reserves of moral authority, infused with defensive insularity.

The rest of the world has not been as consistently grateful for the heroism of 1940 for anywhere near as long as Britain has liked to congratulate itself. And the investment of so much collective pride in one segment of history has consequences for subsequent generations. Canonizing one hour in the past as our finest makes all the ensuing hours drab. It is notable that the most colourful rhetoricians of Brexit belong to the Baby Boom generation or are even younger. Nigel Farage and Boris Johnson were both born in 1964. Jacob Rees-Mogg was born in 1969. He is younger than Kylie Minogue.*

Such is the power of nationalism that it can instil nostalgia for other people's memories. The bank of pride and self-esteem represented by the defeat of Hitler was not deposited by the people who draw on it today for comfort and to dispel their disorientation at Britain's diminished post-imperial status. The Brexit vanguard did not fight the Third Reich, except by proxy in the popular culture of their childhood – the movies, songs and comics that depicted the heroics of the previous generation, sanctified as the supreme imaginable accomplishment. Britain, with some help from Hollywood, made an overbearing parent of its own history, in whose shadow the peacetime progeny felt unable to shine.

Some of those children seem to have carried around a restless craving for battle re-enactment, wanting always to be surviving the Blitz, or sailing small vessels to aid in the evacuation of Dunkirk, or storming a beach in Normandy. The Tory leader who did actually command a battery in the D-Day operation was Ted Heath. His wartime experience made him a passionate advocate of continental cooperation, culminating in his successful campaign to get Britain into the EEC.† The Tory Boomers never forgave him.

---

* This will always be true and never cease to be surprising.

† There is some polling evidence that this distinction pertained even in 2016. While overall there was a correlation between age and voting Leave, with a clear majority of pensioners backing Brexit, within the very oldest segment that had memories of the Second World War, there was a discernible tilt back towards Remain.

Britain's post-war relationship with Europe has been defined not by the veterans of conflict but by the children who idolized them. That is how it evolved into a destabilizing mix of hysteria and complacency; aggression and wounded affront. That is how the peaceful, democratic and law-abiding Europe was cast simultaneously as a harmless joke and a deadly threat to the national way of life. That is why that *Daily Mirror* 'Achtung! Surrender' headline was meant to be funny but not ironic. It is a species of nationalism summarized by the Irish writer Fintan O'Toole as 'a peculiar cocktail of raw xenophobic hysteria, cool intellectual glibness and pure pantomime'.

Pro-Europeans didn't feel any great urgency in responding to that threat because they didn't find it threatening. Liberal opinion was not intimidated by glib nationalism and didn't see how the glibness cloaked something much harder. No great effort went into dismantling silly anti-Europe mythologies or telling rival stories about sovereignty, the national interest and the benefits that EU membership conferred; how Brussels was a place where national power and prestige were amplified, not depleted.

For too long, the Eurosceptic position was treated as a symptom of cultural obsolescence in the Conservative Party. We watched with relish as the Tory vessel capsized and then sank beneath waves of public contempt. We thought their ideological cargo would be lost at sea.

Much of the social and cultural liberalization that occurred through the nineties was permanent. Britain at the start of the new millennium was a more tolerant, less bigoted place than it had been before. David Cameron understood that and forced his party to adapt, or at least to pretend to have adapted. But it was an epic mistake to think that banging on about Europe was a reactionary spasm. It was the beat of a drum in a battle for political control of a national identity, and only one side was fighting seriously. That was the side that eventually won.

The other side, the one that would become the Remainers, wasted years in complacency thinking Euroscepticism was nothing more than the dyspeptic burp of a few fringe-dwelling curmudgeons struggling to digest modernity.

The political muscles that would have made the case for Britain as part of Europe atrophied from lack of use. We realized too late what was at stake. By the time we understood that pro-European Britain was a homeland to defend, it had already been overrun.

Go back to that photograph of me in 1996, with my carefree idiot grin. I had an idea of Britain that was modern for its time, and I fell into the banal trap of youth, thinking that the world would take my modernity as its standard and not make my politics obsolete. I forgot (or was too inexperienced) to consider that political tides can go out as fast as they come in; that I too could end up just like those loonies and fruitcakes, steeped in nostalgia for a country that was lost and never coming back.

CHAPTER 4

JUS SOLI

It is the destiny of the emigrant that the foreign land does not become his homeland: his homeland becomes foreign.

Alfred Polgar

(i) Not cricket

Before I was allowed to work in the parliamentary press gallery, I was vetted for treasonous tendencies. This is a normal security check before issuing an access pass to the Palace of Westminster. They can't trust just anyone to roam the corridors of power unaccompanied. I confirmed that I was not, nor had ever been, a terrorist or conspirator against the government, nor had I knowingly consorted with that kind of person. I also had to supply the Home Office naturalization number that had been issued to my parents, confirming their transition from alien to citizen. They dug out the two faded certificates, dated July 1980, attesting that an oath of loyalty had been sworn to HM Elizabeth II, her heirs and successors.

By a quirk of immigration policy, I was British before my parents. I benefited from *jus soli* – right of soil – the legal entitlement to take on the citizenship of the land in which you are born, an avenue that was closed by the Thatcher government with the 1983 Nationality Act.

Had I been born in the same London hospital a decade later, under the revised rules, I would have entered the world as a South African. I might have acquired the same affection for Britain, but it wouldn't have counted as patriotism until I had taken the oath of allegiance.

Until recently, I did not give much thought to the question of whether my Britishness was a matter of personal preference, an official permission granted or a birthright to be claimed. Immigration rules down the years have shifted the emphasis and changed the frame of that question many times. Partly that is a response to migration patterns, but it is also a barometer of national self-confidence. A country at ease with itself is also more receptive to newcomers.

And the most sensitive questions of political engagement, for migrants and the people into whose midst they migrate, arise at the boundaries of belonging and integration.

Going back once again to the inverse Clausewitz principle – the function of democracy as mediation between different interests – there is a question hidden in that proposition about exactly who qualifies for representation and on what terms. Nationality is not the same as citizenship. And a new identity isn't formed as soon as a new passport is issued. Who gets to arbitrate; who are the gatekeepers of admission to the political community? In the preceding chapters, I have talked about nationhood in terms of *feeling* British. But it is also clear that those feelings depend on the reactions of other people and how those attitudes are then expressed in law.

I never had to declare my loyalty. I did once sit the Life in the

UK Test, an exam on Britishness that was introduced as a necessary qualification for naturalization by the Labour government in 2005. I was researching a feature article on citizenship, which was added to the school curriculum as a mandatory topic around the same time. This was all happening in the long shadow of 9/11 and a great spasm of national anxiety about integration, segregation and what was commonly seen as a stubborn separateness of some Muslim communities that was hothousing fundamentalism and incubating young terrorists.

It was always that way round – failure of the immigrant to integrate, as if it were that easy; as if only laziness, arrogance or cultural backwardness made people cling to the identities they had brought with them from abroad; as if the doors had been flung wide open and only British Muslims, through stubborn quirks of faith and diet, refused to walk through.

I wasn't convinced. But teaching citizenship to everyone, regardless of their background, seemed like a sensible idea in a society that didn't habitually discuss the condition of its democracy or the responsibilities attached to it. There are people whose families go back generations in Britain who might benefit from a refresher course in civics (some of them sit in Parliament).

The utility of the history test was less obvious. I turned up at a tiny internet café on Essex Road in Islington that had been authorized to administer the exam. It was just me and a nervous young Somali man. I gave the best answers I could to multiple-choice questions on topics that ranged from the benefits system to late-medieval history. I had read the official study guide beforehand (being a nerd and unable to contemplate a test without revision) and would probably have failed without it.

I scored 20 out of 24. The pass mark is 18. The test has got harder since then. Sample questions online now ask which county in England hosts Stonehenge and when the Viking Danelaw settlement started. There is no way my parents would have known that in July 1980. I had to google it.

The last part of my enquiry into the naturalization process took me to a citizenship ceremony, which I expected to be sullen and bureaucratic but found quite moving. It took place in a chamber of some municipal grandeur in Lambeth Town Hall. Most of the new Britons were of West African origin. They and their families had dressed properly for the occasion, in Sunday best – suits for the men, big brightly coloured dresses and hats for women. Oaths were sworn on the Bible. Everyone sang 'God Save the Queen'. Applause and hugs followed. Sunlight streamed through the tall windows onto the wooden dais.

Most political arguments around immigration policy in Britain (and most countries that import labour) start from the same common misconception – that loyalty is a zero-sum game. It is the idea that there is a fixed capacity for allegiance in each one of us, and if someone is foreign-born and reserves a portion of attachment to some overseas territory, their commitment to Britain is proportionally diminished. The more the migrant cares about the old country, the less reliable they are as a citizen of the new one.

There is something intuitive in that proposition. National identities are traditionally exclusive and historically defined by conflict with other nations. It was hard to be German *and* British during the First World War, which is why aristocrats descended from the line of 'Sachsen-Coburg und Gotha' rebranded themselves as the House of Windsor. But for many citizens of a modern Western democracy, there is some hybridization in identity. It is impossible to strip us down to a single allegiance without some violence to the soul. The right to retain that hybrid identity isn't something we necessarily notice, except when it is withdrawn.

A clear expression of that zero-sum fallacy was famously provided by Norman Tebbit, a former chairman of the Conservative Party, in a newspaper interview in April 1990. He set Britain's Indian and Pakistani communities a sporting challenge: 'A large proportion of Britain's Asian population fail to pass the cricket test. Which side do they cheer for? It's an interesting test. Are you still harking back to where you came from, or where you are?'

The cricket test, or Tebbit test as it is sometimes known, entered the permanent lexicon of immigration debate. Amid what is wrong with it, there is a banal truth. Sport reveals emotional attachment. My parents will never feel their guts contract in the dying minutes of extra time in an England football fixture, knowing that a penalty shoot-out is coming. They probably wouldn't even know there was a game on. I find it so stressful, I can hardly be in the room. That might be one way to measure the gap between first and second generations, but it isn't a precision tool.

The Tebbit test touches on another, more interesting truth: national identity, like sporting fandom, is as much about alignment with a narrative as it is about material facts. Obviously, action on the pitch is happening in the real world. Actual balls fly into real goals. But the power of the result to change your mood, to bring elation or despair, comes from the extent to which you have projected yourself onto a group of strangers who happen to be wearing the colours that represent a particular place. From a purely rational perspective, it is nonsense when football fans use the first-person plural to describe performance on the pitch – '*we* were rubbish in defence/*we* were robbed of a penalty'. The speaker has no meaningful agency over the outcome. But that 'we' describes participation not in the match but in the *journey* – the sequence of victories and defeats through time – and there the first person plural is correct. The longer the fan has followed the team, the more memories have been amassed of great players from the past, trophies won and managers sacked, the more emotion has been invested in the journey and the stronger 'we' will feel.

When it comes to national allegiance, it takes time for an immigrant to become part of that 'we' if you aren't born and raised in it. It is a private and intimate process. You start out as a character in a story you have inherited about the place you are from, and then you have to write that person into a new plot line in a new location. You feel as if you are climbing on board a moving vehicle having missed the start of the journey when the other passengers were getting to know each other. Everyone else on the bus knows all the chants. You have to try to pick up the words, despite only having boarded at a motorway service station a few minutes ago when the rest of the crowd has been singing since breakfast.

One thing that is guaranteed to slow the process, or send it into reverse, is a loyalty test. It is being told you are getting it wrong by some self-appointed arbiter of the club rules. It is being scolded by the old-timers because your singing isn't loud enough, because you haven't put in the hard yards and haven't earned the right to wear the shirt. It is being told that, despite your claim to support the team, you aren't a *proper* fan.

The loyalty test isn't exclusive to nationalists or right-wing politics. There is a scene captured on video of Jeremy Corbyn, then just a backbench MP, speaking at an event in 2013. He referred to an incident in which Jewish members of an audience had confronted the Palestinian envoy to the UK about comments he had made, except Corbyn didn't say 'Jewish', he said 'Zionist'. Their interventions, he explained, exposed two problems: 'One is that they don't want to study history and secondly, having lived in this country for a very long time, probably all their lives, they don't understand English irony either.'

The implication is that Jews who recognize the claim of Israel as a national homeland automatically forfeit part of their claim to be truly English. Their fixed allocation of loyalty is divided. Corbynism never asserted that Jews were barred from the movement. It just made it clear that Jews could not be good socialists and also Zionist. They had to pick a side. That was their cricket test, although they would claim – without a hint of English irony – to have nothing in common with the politics of Norman Tebbit.

(ii) Breaking point

On the morning of 16 June 2016, Thomas Mair left the small semi-detached brick house on a quiet suburban street in Birstall, West Yorkshire, where he lived alone with a neatly arranged stock of tinned foods – baked beans, evaporated milk, strawberries in syrup – and a fastidiously curated collection of Nazi memorabilia. Carrying a Tesco bag and a black holdall, he boarded a bus to Birstall market square. There he loitered. He ate a Flake. He binned the wrapper. He took up a position near the local library, which was due to be visited by Jo Cox, the local Labour MP. When Cox arrived shortly before 1 p.m., Mair approached her, shot her at close range three times and stabbed her repeatedly. 'This is for Britain,' he said as the knife went in. Also, according to witnesses, 'Keep Britain independent' and 'Put Britain first.'

Mair fled the scene but was soon tracked down by police. 'I'm a political activist,' he told the arresting officer. He was not a member of any far-right organizations. He had taught himself the doctrines of white supremacism alone at home, from mail-order fascist publications, and in the library. He was (and from his jail cell presumably still is) convinced that liberal and left-wing politicians promoted immigration and multiculturalism. They did this, he believed, in order to dilute the ethnic purity of his kindred folk, making the white race weak and easier to manipulate. Once he had discovered this threat, Mair recruited himself as a warrior for the defence of the nation. Jo Cox, as a passionate advocate for remaining in the EU, was his enemy. In court, when asked to identify himself, he declared: 'My name is "death to traitors, freedom for Britain".'

A week after Jo Cox's murder, in the early hours of 24 June, as it became clear that the referendum on EU membership had been won by the Leavers, Nigel Farage addressed a rally in London. The result, he said, was 'a victory for real people, a victory for ordinary people, a victory for decent people'. It was achieved, he added, 'without a single shot being fired'.

Farage had forgotten the shots that were fired into Jo Cox, or more likely didn't count them as part of the referendum campaign. Mair was not a member of any party or pro-Brexit group. He had no friends or relationships. He slotted into a ready media template – the disturbed loner; the isolated maniac. But he had also researched Jo Cox's life and her political beliefs, printing out pro-European articles she had published online and storing them in his library alongside items about Anders Breivik, a Norwegian white supremacist who had killed 77 people in July 2011. Mair was charged and convicted of terrorism offences.

The police officer leading the investigation into Cox's killing believed that the referendum campaign was an aggravating factor, or at least that the febrile atmosphere around the campaign had made a difference, tipping Mair's mental state from seething introspection to something more proactive. 'Brexit did play a part,' Detective Superintendent Nick Wallen told a BBC documentary after Mair's trial. 'The country was divided, so that played a part in tensions within the community.'

But 17.4 million people voted for Brexit; 52 per cent of everyone who expressed a view. It would be grotesque to imply that their choice contained any moral complicity with Mair's agenda. The point is rather that Jo Cox's killer was a volatile particle at the outermost periphery of the vast and furious miasma.

Thomas Mair's paranoid derangement was the refined and deadliest iteration of a mainstream nationalist proposition at the heart of the Brexit campaign – that nationhood itself was at stake; that something essential about what it meant to be Britain had been surrendered to foreigners; that it needed reclaiming.

In September 2015, when the referendum was planned but not yet declared, Farage rallied his UK Independence Party with the prospect of 'a once in a lifetime opportunity to get back the independence and self-government of this nation'. Addressing an audience of mostly middle-aged and older white men, he continued: 'Our message is clear: we want our country back.' When the campaign got under way, that slogan was painted across the purple open-topped battle bus that carried Farage to his target voters. *We Want Our Country Back.*

Back from whom?

The morning of the Cox assassination, Farage, as head of the Leave.EU campaign, had unveiled a poster with the slogan 'Breaking Point'. It showed a dense crowd of refugees trailing back as far as the eye could see. There was not a white face in the throng. The message was plain: EU membership was the pipeline channelling ethnic interlopers into Britain, which was now full to bursting. Boris Johnson held his nose in affected distaste. 'Not our campaign,' he said. 'Not my politics.'

It *was* his politics.* His Vote Leave campaign (the official pro-Brexit group) had its own variant of the same poster. It proclaimed: 'Turkey (population 76 million) is joining the EU.' The parable of national pollution was depicted as a trail of dirty footprints entering an open British passport. (Turkey was notionally a candidate for EU membership but that was an obsolescent ambition in 2016.)

---

* Johnson's attitude to race is not straightforward. As Mayor of London he affected liberal stances, even endorsing in theory (but never implementing) an amnesty for illegal immigrants. But his back catalogue of *Daily Telegraph* columns is peppered with casual prejudice: African children as 'piccaninnies' with 'watermelon smiles'; veiled Muslim women resembling letter boxes. The way to make sense of the contradictions is that he could, absent other pressures, be liberal-minded on many things. But in the event that personal ambition forced him to choose between principled liberalism and cynical self-advancement by means of coarse nationalism, he wouldn't hesitate to wallow in the latter.

Plenty of Conservative enthusiasts for Brexit claimed to be unhappy with the racist undertones of the campaign, although they managed to keep those qualms in check until long after the polls closed. For a certain kind of high-minded Tory Euro-sceptic, the demand for sovereignty should not be sullied by explicit associations with racial homogeneity. They wanted to be seen as liberal-minded enthusiasts for free trade (although not via the EU single market). All the talk of immigration control was consistent with their ambitions but offended them by its vulgarity. They liked the votes that Farage's methods could bring in but, mindful of their party's stately facade, preferred to take delivery at the tradesmen's entrance.

In the days after the referendum, I started to hear stories of casual discrimination and aggression against people whose skin tone marked them out as a potential foreigner. Friends and colleagues were told by strangers in the street or leaning out of passing cars that they should go back where they had come from. Mostly they had come from London, but that wasn't what their verbal assailants had in mind.

There is some evidence of a spike in racially motivated hate crime in the aftermath of the Brexit vote, although these things are hard to measure because not every victim tells the police. According to a study by researchers at the University of Bath, the volume went up by 15–25 per cent in the three months after the referendum compared to the previous period, but settled down again not long after. That amounts to around 2,000 extra incidents. The authors of the study surmise that victory for the Leave side led to a short but intense suspension of the social norms that had previously kept certain racist behaviours in check.

People who had previously wished that immigrants would 'go home' but felt a prohibition on telling them so to their faces, read the national vote for Brexit as a dissolution of that taboo.

The project of taking Britain out of the EU was not primarily or consciously devised as a racist enterprise, nor even conceived with explicit intent to narrow criteria for belonging to the nation. Brexit was a political revolution that appealed to a diverse electorate for complex reasons that will be examined later.

But the campaign effected a paradigm change in the way British politics dealt with questions of national identity. It was nationalist in character – mobilizing all the myths of heroic collective destiny, foreign oppression, the golden age that would be revived on liberation noted in Chapter 2. The potential for the whole business to degenerate into a vast loyalty test was intrinsic to its nationalism.

If the nation is on a mission, those who oppose the mission are the enemy. The mission is never complete because the idea of the nation that fires the nationalist imagination doesn't correspond to reality. And so that unavailable ideal nation will always need taking back from *someone*.

(iii) On the banks of the Tiber

Before Brexit, by far the most famous expression of fear that mass migration could be the undoing of a nation was the prophecy that Enoch Powell made in a speech on 20 April 1968. The Conservative shadow Defence Secretary told his audience in Birmingham that Britain was 'heaping up its own funeral pyre' by allowing too many Commonwealth citizens to settle in the country; that his white constituents 'found themselves made strangers in their own country'.

He predicted that 'the black man will have the whip hand over the white man.' His peroration cited the verse from Virgil by which the whole speech came to be known: 'Like the Roman, I seem to see "the River Tiber foaming with much blood".'

The Tory leader at the time, Ted Heath, thought the message was 'racialist in tone and liable to exacerbate racial tensions'. Powell was sacked from the front bench and enjoyed the status of a martyr for his radical right-wing opinion on immigration.

The 'Rivers of Blood' speech also set an informal parameter for what constituted civilized mainstream debate on race and integration. To be compared to Powell was a mark of having crossed the line. There was much rhetorical paddling in the shallow end of the Tiber over the ensuing decades, but anyone who wanted a career in Parliament knew not to stir up the foam.

Although complaints about migration volumes were a perennial feature of politics, the numbers involved were stable through the seventies and eighties. There were many years when Britain was a net exporter of people. From the mid nineties onwards, there were net inflows – a measure of economic buoyancy and globalization gathering pace. There was a steep uptick after 2004, when 10 new members, including relatively poor former communist countries, were admitted to the EU. (There was also a dip after the 2008 financial crisis.) In the period 1991–95, the annual average net increase in UK population from migration was 37,000, according to House of Commons library research. By the second half of the noughties (when Brexit was being debated), that figure had risen to 266,000.

The numbers can only ever be a rough indicator. The counting process is imprecise and official methods change. In political debate, it doesn't help that the catch-all term 'immigrant' is used for people arriving in Britain with a variety of motives from diverse places: penniless refugees from war zones and bankers hopping from one global financial hub to another. When people complain that our little North Atlantic island is getting overcrowded or that jobs are being taken by undeserving foreigners, they generally don't mean white Australians.

New Labour was particularly incoherent when it came to immigration. The Blair government's enthusiastic embrace of EU enlargement was a dramatic gesture of open-door liberalism, but it came against a backdrop of neuralgic rhetoric against 'bogus' asylum seekers, alleged to be 'swamping' public services and, in Blair's own words, 'playing the system'. In the decade between 1997 and 2007, there were five migration-related bills. The advertised quality of new measures was always toughness.

The Cameron government took up the same cudgel, promising to cut the overall level of immigration year on year. The target was never met. As had been the pattern under New Labour, the draconian rhetoric combined with continued inflows of people made a toxic cocktail. It broadcast simultaneously the messages that immigration was a curse and that there was nothing politicians could do about it.

The tone of government policy implied that a foreigner intending to settle in Britain probably had nefarious intent, and that there was a whiff of something illicit about those who were here already. In case anyone missed the point, Farage was always nearby to spell it out. 'Any normal and fair-minded person would have a perfect right to be concerned if a group of Romanian people suddenly moved in next door,' he said, to a minor flurry of mainstream opprobrium in 2014.

A year earlier, the Home Office had run a pilot scheme for a public information campaign aimed at undocumented migrants. Known internally as 'Operation Vaken', it formed part of an official strategy to drive down migration numbers by making Britain a 'hostile environment' for anyone not legally entitled to residency. Billboard vans were driven around parts of London with a high density of foreign-born residents with the warning: 'Go home or face arrest.' Even Farage, in a feint of moderation, called the campaign 'unpleasant'. It was scrapped. It was not the intent of the policy that broke a taboo, there being nothing unusual in another crackdown on illegal immigration. It was the instruction to *go home*, which sounded like the tearing down of a fence that had once marked the boundary between mainstream government ambition and the hooligan harrying of strangers in the street.

By a process of mission creep and institutional vindictiveness, the Home Office 'hostile environment' turned a bureaucracy for processing migration status into an instrument of propaganda and ultimately persecution. Thousands of people of Caribbean origin, the 'Windrush generation' that had been invited to settle in the UK to fill labour shortages after the Second World War, were harassed, interned and deported. There was no doubt that they were legally and morally entitled to British citizenship, but they didn't necessarily have documents to prove it after so many decades of not being asked.

Here was a new and sinister development in immigration policy. A lifetime of belonging in Britain – as a matter of culture, self-identification and law – was irrelevant to a state that decided to withdraw the right to be British. The Home Secretary behind the hostile environment policy was Theresa May, and it was not surprising when she became prime minister in July 2016 (having desultorily supported the Remain side in the referendum) that she interpreted her mandate exclusively in terms of border control and migration.

She did not have any other way of defining the task. When asked what the terms of Britain's withdrawal from the EU would be, she would say only, 'Brexit means Brexit.' When pressed for embellishment, she added the national colours, saying it would be a 'red, white and blue Brexit'.

It became clear later in the year, when May gave her first keynote speech to the Tories' annual conference, that the priority – the axiom of a proper Brexit – was ending the automatic entitlement of EU citizens to live and work in the UK.* (Freedom of movement within the bloc had been a reciprocal right, but the idea that curtailing it might also be a debilitation of powers attached to a British passport was alien to the Eurosceptics and poorly explained by pro-Europeans.)

Ending free movement also involved a conceptual innovation in UK immigration policy – retroactively changing the status of people who had settled in the country on terms that they thought were fixed in perpetuity. There were at least three million EU nationals living in Britain, and they had not

---

* May's fixation on this point was so complete that she did not even realize that ending free movement necessitated also complete withdrawal from the EU single market. She had to have that consequence of the announcement she had just made explained to her by an official once the speech had already been delivered.

conceived of themselves as aliens in the way that Brexit suddenly cast them. Their migration had been internal to the European space. Now Britain was declaring that category invalid in the concentric circles of belonging. You could be European or British, but not both.

If you were French, German, Polish, Slovak, but had lived in Britain for years, worked there, fallen in love, married, had children, sent them to a local school, Brexit made you reapply to be somewhere you thought you were already – home.

You didn't have to be directly targeted by the policy to feel it as an aggression against the idea of a hybrid identity. I felt it like a rough fingernail picking at the seam where the fabrics of belonging, the different stories I could tell about who I was and where I had come from, were joined.

When the mood against migration had hardened in the past, the change was expressed in law to be applied for new arrivals. The 1983 Nationalities Act, for example, made it harder for a hypothetical younger version of me to be British. It didn't reach back in time and snatch away citizenship status that the real me had owned since birth.

(iv) Citizens of Remainia

The speech in which May made aliens of the Europeans living in Britain at the time also alienated a much wider audience. The lines that did it were these:

Today, too many people in positions of power behave as though they have more in common with international elites than with the people down the road, the people they employ, the people they pass in the street. But if you believe you're a citizen of the world, you're a citizen of nowhere. You don't understand what the very word 'citizenship' means.

I was watching that speech in Birmingham and flinched at the words 'citizen of nowhere'. They belonged to a sinister ideological tradition, with strands on the extreme left and right. Stalin had run a paranoid campaign against 'rootless cosmopolitans' – a euphemism for Jews – whose cross-border cultural attachments were deemed inherently incompatible with loyalty to the Soviet motherland. Hitler had also denounced cosmopolitanism as a symptom of moral degeneracy. 'Globalist' is a code word that communicates the same idea in the modern constellations of white supremacism and loosely affiliated conspiracy theorists.

May's advisers assured me that those unfortunate echoes were accidental; that the speech had not been a dog-whistle summons to the nastiest subsection of the Brexit-voting cohort. And May was certainly tin-eared on other things enough that she wouldn't have caught the resonance herself. In any case, 'citizen of nowhere' became a badge of honour for people who felt driven into a state of emotional exile by the referendum campaign and its aftermath – those of us who had an idea of the open, tolerant, liberal-minded country we lived in, the island of Remainia, and saw it sinking into the sea.

Maybe that place had been a fantasy all along, or more accurately, an imagined community fashioned from only half of the nation. Leavonia, the other half, had a very different story to tell about its origins and its future.

That schism accounts for a lot of conflict and misunderstanding over what the word 'Brexit' even means. The fault line existed long before the referendum, but beneath the party-political crust, tectonic plates, moved by the slow-roiling magma of social and economic change across generations, were readying the ground for an eruption.

That process has been best described in *Brexitland*, by Maria Sobolewska and Robert Ford. As the authors observe:

> The EU Referendum itself was not so much a moment of creation, but rather a moment of awakening: a moment when the social and political processes long underway finally became obvious, and the different groups of voters finally recognized themselves as two distinct and opposed camps.

A significant part of that revealed polarization was demographic sorting – the coalescence of like-minded tribes in distinct neighbourhoods, accelerated by the pattern of young people leaving their home towns to go to university and never returning. Some cities became cosmopolitan engines of globalization. Small towns and parts of the countryside were, to use a phrase that became the analytic staple in commentary of the phenomenon, left behind. As Sobolewska and Ford put it:

> Graduates mainly live among other graduates, in ethnically diverse places that accord with, and reinforce, their belief in a dynamic and diverse Britain. White voters with low education levels also live around similar people, in ageing and declining places which accord with, and reinforce, their sense of marginalization and stagnation.

My home town of Brighton has two universities. It attracts

young professionals in creative industries and provides a lot of commuter traffic back and forth from London. It is also one of the most densely pro-European parts of the land. People flew EU flags from their windows during the campaign. Some still do. If the vote had been limited to our city, the result would have been 75 per cent for Remain. Judging by local council data, eight in every ten of my near neighbours were Remainers. There were symmetrical imbalances all over the country. Skegness, a less prosperous seaside town, in the east of England, wanted to quit Europe as much as Brighton wanted to stay.

It is absurd to imagine that the referendum result allocated people to one of two neatly drawn reservations – a metropolitan citadel fortified with vegan cafés, and a provincial hinterland patrolled by white vans flying the St George's Cross. Clearly, it is more nuanced than that.

It is also risky to infer much about British attitudes to race from that result. The trends on that front are disputed and hard to measure in opinion polls. A steady fall in the proportion of people saying they hold racist attitudes (which is the broad pattern measured since the 1980s)* probably reflects a genuine decline in racism alongside growing awareness among racists that their views are not something to admit to holding. The potency of that taboo might produce a climate in which there are fewer racists but a more assertive, defiant strain of racism in that minority.

Where race fits into discussion of immigration policy is an

---

* For example, between 1983 and 1996, the annual British Social Attitudes survey asked people how unhappy they would be if a family member married someone black or Asian. The figure was around 50 per cent in the eighties and dropped to around 35 per cent by the mid nineties.

even trickier question. Not everyone who thinks borders should be policed is a racist, but every racist thinks borders are not tightly enough controlled.

In the years immediately after Brexit, immigration dropped below other concerns when voters were asked to list their priorities, suggesting that withdrawal from the EU satisfied some of that grievance. That didn't mean it couldn't be whipped up again. Farage's satisfaction at the referendum result was predictably short-lived. He was soon to be seen on the Kent coast, invigilating national whiteness at the Cliffs of Dover, complaining about the porous maritime boundary where migrants on small vessels could come ashore unimpeded. In response to that challenge, Boris Johnson's government cooked up cruel, cockamamie schemes to drive the boats back to France or deport their passengers to a processing centre in Rwanda.

It is hard to argue that Tory Euroscepticism is an exclusively racist doctrine when its enactment as policy has coincided with so much ethnic diversity at the top of British politics. Britain's first post-EU cabinet was the most multiracial in the country's history. In recent years, the Treasury has been run by Chancellors of Pakistani, Indian, Iraqi Kurdish and Ghanaian heritage.* The Home Office and Foreign Office portfolios have regularly been held by men and women of colour. The third post-Brexit prime minister, incumbent at the time of writing, is a second-generation Indian immigrant.

Rishi Sunak's arrival in Downing Street was a rebuke to the

---

* Sajid Javid, Rishi Sunak, Nadhim Zahawi, Kwasi Kwarteng. It is worth adding that three of those served in a single year. When you replace ministers that often, there is more opportunity for diverse appointments, but it isn't a given.

school of left-liberal commentary that orients itself in debates about race and immigration using irredeemable Tory bigotry as a fixed compass point. The reality is more complicated. Social conservatism, often with a religious component, is a feature of many immigrant communities that aligns them more naturally with the Conservative party than Labour.

The same applies to the ethos of individual enterprise and economic self-reliance that drives many immigrant success stories. Powell and his acolytes cast a long shadow that still deters many immigrants and their children who might otherwise be attracted to Tory policy, but the effect has waned over time. (And it certainly won't be restored by complaints on the left that prominent Conservative ministers of African or Asian heritage are somehow deficient in racial consciousness or forfeit their minority status by alignment with the party of white privilege.*)

No other European country has a matching record of ethnic diversity in its most senior political offices. Parties of the far right, ethnic exceptionalism and anti-liberalism are well enough represented in continental governments to shake pro-Europeans out of any romantic notion that EU membership is inoculation against ultra-nationalist politics.

Ethnic diversity in the cabinet didn't have any measurable impact in liberalizing migration policy in the Conservative party. After Brexit, the nationalist caucus that had fixated on

---

* In September 2022, Rupa Huq, a Labour MP, was suspended from the parliamentary party and apologized for describing Kwasi Kwarteng, then Chancellor, as 'superficially black', the inference being that party allegiance trumps pigmentation in any political taxonomy of racial identity. Sunak's arrival in Downing Street elicited much of the same cognitive distress among some leftwing commentators.

EU membership as the prop holding the country's doors open to all and sundry railed instead against the dreaded flotilla of dinghies carrying interlopers across the Channel. In November 2022, the Home Secretary, Suella Braverman, told the House of Commons that Britain was facing an 'invasion' by people who were only pretending to be refugees.

To liberal ears, there was a grating dissonance between that rhetoric and Braverman's own status as a second-generation migrant. The same dismay was stirred by Braverman's equally strident predecessor at the Home Office, Priti Patel, and a generation earlier by Michael Howard, a Jewish Home Secretary. The complaint, in these instances, is that settled immigrants and their offspring ought to be more sensitive to the needs of new arrivals, which is another way of saying they should be more grateful to the liberalism of previous regimes for giving them the space to become conservative. It is a glib argument, building a hypocrisy out of someone's personal circumstances to invalidate their politics. At worst, it swerves into a discreet leftwing racism, the implication being that people of colour have some debt of allegiance to the political tribe that claims ownership of anti-racism. It is a variant of the loyalty test.

There are many good reasons to dislike immigration policy and rhetoric when they are vindictive and ineffective, but the birthplace of a minister's parents isn't relevant to that evaluation. Migrants are entitled to be nationalists and opponents of nationalism won't win their arguments by claiming that skin colour is a disqualification from holding certain opinions. Race is frequently inseparable from discussions of nationalism but it can also be a distraction. The nationalist's target is outsiders, *the others*, where race is only one available denomination.

How much racism was there in Brexit itself? Enough to radicalize liberal Remainers in their objections to it. And the expression of that aversion aggravated Leavers who felt strongly that their motives were more noble. That dynamic accelerated another vicious polarizing cycle. Pro-Europeans saw themselves as defenders of liberal civilization under siege by nationalist maniacs, which felt like sufficient moral imperative to decide that the result of the referendum should be overturned. That resistance confirmed a pro-Brexit account of Remain as a creed of snooty metropolitan liberals who dismissed provincial Britain as a barbarian wasteland.

I have felt the years since the referendum as a time when politics was captured by nationalism – and for the reasons described in this and previous chapters, I experienced that as a state of emotional and psychological exile. But to make sense of post-Brexit politics I have to recognize that exile was a condition of the other side too. Each tribe felt despised by the other. Each was competing to get its country back. It is possible, and I think necessary, to acknowledge that symmetry. That is hard when the losing side sees most of its arguments from the referendum vindicated by subsequent events, and feels perpetually cheated as a result. It takes a leap of empathy to recognize parity of emotional investment in the two opposing positions, separate from the historical argument about which campaign dealt more in facts and which relied on prejudice.

People who have never migrated anywhere can still feel dramatic social, cultural and economic change as a kind of disenfranchisement – a redefinition of their homeland on terms that make them feel less at home. That dismay will sometimes express itself as racism. It is a recoil from difference, with racial differences often being most conspicuous and the ones on which campaigning politics can gain the firmest purchase. That doesn't mean race is the irreducible core of the disagreement.

The impulse to be suspicious of people who are unlike ourselves is innately human. That isn't a fatalistic observation. Politics can be a process of minimizing the suspicion by illuminating the things we have in common. The differences do not have to be treated as a raw material of fear to be mined for electoral gain. The politicians who are most skilled in that industry are also the ones least qualified to manage effective government and least trustworthy as custodians of democracy.

There is also a mode of anti-populist politics that is marked by a more subtle kind of intolerance – an eye-rolling impatience with retrograde ideas that comes across as a demand that the hoodwinked electorate get real; get with the liberal programme. That also fails.

People who have an emotional attachment to their idea of a homeland do not want to be told that it is an irrational fiction. Everyone sometimes uses nostalgia as analgesia against the present. No one wants to be written off as a pitiful junky, blotting out the pain of obsolescence and defeat in a brave new world. That caricature inflamed the bitterness of cultural conservatives in the heyday of globalization, and it salts the wounds of liberals today.

There is a difficult line to tread between the requirement of empathy and the trap of appeasement. Nationalist politicians use inflammatory rhetoric to bate their opponents into reactions that can then be used as evidence of cosmopolitan arrogance. It is exhausting trying to navigate that trap. Should liberals bite their tongues for fear that moral outrage at xenophobic language fertilizes more bigotry? That is a formula for acquiescence.

There is a way to break the cycle of mutually reinforcing exile. It involves all of us recognizing that none of us is getting our mythical old country back. There is common ground in the mutual feelings of disorientation and loss. Whether that shared experience is foundation enough for a new national myth of reconciliation will depend on the narrative capabilities of the politicians who want it to be true. There is a story there to be told and, I believe, an audience willing to hear it.

Part Two

HYPERTENSION

CHAPTER 5

THE POTEMKIN SYNDROME

All the world is not, of course, a stage but the crucial ways in which it isn't are not easy to specify.

Erving Goffman

(i) Lessons from a broken laboratory

'Do you see that post over there?' The young soldier pointed his cigarette at an indistinct bump on the other side of the road far beyond the high barbed-wire fence, blending into the dusk. 'If that was a man, I could take him down from here.'

I nodded to show that I understood what an impressive display of sharp-shooting that would be, while hoping not to signal that I approved of killing in cold blood at any range. Also, maybe it was an easy shot for a professional sniper. How would I know?

Was it hard? I asked.

'Like anything else, it takes practice.'

I meant shooting someone, pulling the trigger to eliminate another human being. Was that hard?

'The same. Only hard at first.'

We were idly smoking outside the canteen of a military camp

in northern Chechnya. It was March 2003, during what is generally called the Second Chechen War, although there had been no peaceful interlude since the first one a decade earlier. There was just one long, grinding effort by the Kremlin to suffocate rebellion in the Caucasus republic.

Grozny, the capital, was in ruins from savage assaults by Russian tanks and artillery. The streets into the city were lined with charred concrete crusts, derelict buildings without roofs and apartment blocks missing whole sides; windows blasted glassless. Sometimes the only way to tell the difference between heaps of rubble and family homes was the words 'people live here' sprayed on the remnants of exterior walls.

I had no idea how accurately my new companion could shoot, but his eyes gave me confidence that he was an experienced killer. They were grey-blue, hyper-alert, but eerily lacking a glint. It was a look that measured you without empathy, desensitized to cruelty. I had seen it often in Russia. I had lived there as a student in the mid-nineties. By 2003, I was based in Moscow as a foreign correspondent. I had not planned to spend time in war zones. My reporting beat was business, the transition from a communist economy to a free-market capitalist one. There were plenty of armed thugs on that scene too. The privatization of Russia's natural resources and industrial assets was wholly corrupt and sometimes completed at gunpoint. If you spent any time around the new class of 'businessmen', or went to the clubs where they sat in corners watching other people dance, you met a lot of heavies with paramilitary protection and cold blood in their eyes.

It was unnerving when those eyes stared at you with lethal intent. It happened to me only once, in Nizhny Novgorod, an industrial city 260 miles east of Moscow. I was with a friend, also British, in a café having breakfast. We were approached by two men, shaven-headed, with flattened features as if pressed between two panes of glass, and glintless eyes like the sniper in Grozny. They insisted that we drink some vodka with them. It was around 11 o'clock in the morning. The men wanted to know our reasons for visiting Nizhny Novgorod, and our answers, for reasons I didn't fathom, were unsatisfactory. The conversation became an interrogation, culminating in a demand that we hand over our passports. We refused, at which point it was decided that we should leave the café and the city on pain of death. The exact words, as I recall, were: 'If we ever see you in this town again, we will get someone to break your arms and legs, fuck you up the arse and *then* kill you.'*

Not every small-time crook was hostile to foreigners. On one long cross-country train journey I shared a carriage with a low-ranking hoodlum who also insisted on vodka, but in a spirit of international comradeship. After a few drinks, he was so moved by my interest in his homeland that he offered me a business card and promised to eliminate anyone who dared to get in the way of my future journalistic enquiries.

It didn't take many encounters of that kind to understand why democracy had not caught on in Russia. Throughout the nineties, I watched the chaotic experiment in democracy fizzle and sputter under Boris Yeltsin. Then I saw Vladimir Putin take over the laboratory, abandon the experiment, fake the results and shatter the apparatus. That is how I ended up on an army

---

* I did subsequently visit Nizhny Novgorod several years later, to report on a car factory privatization, but I didn't stay for long.

base learning how much easier killing gets the more you do it.

Putin had come to power in 2000, promising to restore order and national dignity. To prove the point, he pacified Chechnya and propped up a locally recruited, pro-Kremlin administration. To show how grateful Chechens were for their pacification, there was to be a referendum on a new constitution for the republic, confirming that it was 'inseparable' from the Russian motherland. The ruin of Grozny was to be the model for absorption into Russia for people who refused their first invitation. It was the harbinger that stalked Ukrainian cities when Putin ordered their capture two decades later.

He expected a swift victory, with barely a shot fired. It didn't even qualify as a war in the official vocabulary. It was a 'special military operation'. Ukraine was not really a nation in its own right in the Kremlin view. Its people, a Slavic subset of Russians, would welcome Putin's soldiers as liberators, come to dispose of a drug-addled neo-Nazi junta that ruled without popular consent in Kyiv. When it turned out that Ukrainians did in fact have a national identity and that they resisted foreign attack with patriotic ardour, Russian forces adopted a new strategy. The only method of urban warfare they knew was the one previously deployed in Chechnya (and again in Syria, where Russia intervened to support President Assad). The technique was to rain indiscriminate murder onto civilian populations, making it clear that the only options were surrender or death – 'Groznification'.

There is a hindsight bias that views Russia's dalliance with democracy in the nineties as a staging post on the inevitable reversion to neo-Soviet tyranny. Putin did a thorough job persuading many Russians that their culture and history were antithetical to the liberal, effeminate decadence that polluted Western souls so deeply that they had Pride marches instead of military parades. It is the vanity of all dictators to trace their ascent in recent history as an arc of national destiny. But the failure of Russia's experiment in democracy was a more complex and collaborative effort between corrupt politicians in Moscow and complacent Western governments who were happy to see the country's wealth-generating engines handed over to gangsters if it meant they wouldn't fall back into communist hands. It turned out that communists and gangsters could reach an accommodation without having to go via democracy.

I learned a lot of things in Russia, besides how to down 100 millilitres of bootleg vodka without flinching. I came to appreciate how intimately political systems express national cultures, but also how nationalists manipulate that relationship to claim that systems for admitting liberal dissent are alien. I got to know the conditions in which a society comes to prefer authoritarian control to pluralism: how the depletion of the will to uphold democracy starts with a corrosion of confidence that people in power act from motives other than self-enrichment; how it is accelerated when truth becomes a battleground and official information is a weapon of coercion; how it is completed in a state of pervasive, nervous stress, where a sequence of cascading crises blur into a unified chronic state of political hypertension.

I travelled to Grozny in a press convoy with a military escort, by special invitation of the Russian foreign ministry. We were there to witness a new constitutional order rising like a phoenix from the ashes of war. We spent a night on the army base and the next morning travelled by bus to a polling station. It was set up in the large open foyer of a Soviet-era municipal administration building. There was a long trestle table at one end of the room where bored officials sat behind ballot boxes and unused papers. There was tea for the visitors, and bunting to add a dash of festivity. Jaunty music played. Nothing about the scene felt spontaneous or natural. It was a Potemkin village in the country that invented the concept.

The story, dating from the eighteenth century, tells of Catherine II touring newly conquered territory in Crimea, where her favourite military commander, courtier and lover, Grigory Potemkin, hired or forced peasants to play the part of happy villagers on the banks of the River Dnieper. The scene, in front of makeshift huts, would be performed in one location, then disassembled and reassembled further along the shore so the same crew could simulate multiple villages. Historians have cast doubt on the story. It is probably a myth, grown from some seed of truth. Catherine wanted good news, and sycophants would go to elaborate lengths to satisfy her. The Potemkin village caught on in the international lexicon to describe a timeless feature of human nature – power's vanity in wanting to believe that the powerless are grateful for their subordination.

A shortage of voters spoiled the initial effect of the Potemkin village I saw in Grozny. The electorate was on its way, we were told. It was still early. Eventually, as promised, a steady stream of electors started to flow in in fulfilment of their civic duty. Some said they had voted for the new constitution; others preferred to say nothing. The result came through that evening, before ballots in remote areas could feasibly have been counted: 96 per cent were in favour of the new constitution on a turnout of 80 per cent. Putin said he had expected a good result but that the numbers 'surpassed even our most optimistic expectations'.

In September 2022, the Kremlin engineered Potemkin referendums in four partially occupied regions of eastern Ukraine. There was no realistic prospect of a fair ballot, nor much serious pretence at organizing one. Much of the population had fled in terror. Some who remained voted at gunpoint. The declared official results ranged from 96 per cent to 99 per cent in favour of annexation by Moscow. In towns nearby, where the occupying Russian army had been driven back by Ukrainian forces, hundreds of bodies were being uncovered in mass graves.

(ii) Trust deficiency disorder

It is easy to forget that Russia had better options than murderous kleptocracy when the Soviet Union collapsed in 1991. It would have been naive to expect parliamentary democracy to spring up like mushrooms after rain, but there was nothing imaginary about the aspiration of ordinary Russians to swap repressive single-party rule for a system that respected human rights and held fair elections.

Watching that aspiration die at close quarters was important to my political education, because it was the first time I felt viscerally repelled by politics. I also started to find journalism demoralizing. The walls that held the truth back from us were too high and fiercely guarded for me to scale. Better reporters, with more courage and stamina than me, managed the task. I quit not long after that trip to Chechnya.

Much of Putin's appeal to Russians, especially out in the vast sprawling provinces, was an end to capricious, arbitrary power and its replacement with dependable authority. Appeals to democratic principle don't have much traction when political freedom comes as a bundle with constant fear of criminal violence.

Britain has not experienced anything like the descent into lawlessness that Russians lived through in the nineties. But when you see a democracy wither and die on foreign ground, you end up wondering how deep the roots really go in your native land; whether there is something in the climate and soil that keeps it hardy and how prolonged a spell of bad weather might have to be for the harvest to fail.

Britain and Russia have features in common, but the parallel lines are separated by a lot of historical and cultural difference. The two countries are sometimes described as matching bookends on the opposite sides of Europe. Both are geographically destined to be involved in the continent's business while persuaded also that their national destiny makes them something other than just European. (Russia has its vast Asian hinterland; the UK has its obsession with the Atlantic, the 'special relationship' with America, memories of a globe-straddling colonial heyday.) Both have struggled with the loss of superpower status – Britain is still shaking off delusions of imperial grandeur; Russia is resentful of its post-Cold War relegation from the geopolitical premier league. But Britain's representative institutions have evolved over hundreds of years, during which period Russia's default setting has been autocracy.

It is possible that I load more weight on the comparison than it can bear because I spent so many years shuttling between the two countries as their relationship swerved from enmity to intimacy and back again. Why did democracy work in one place and not the other? What would it have taken for the positive traits of the British system to catch on in Russia, and what would it take to cultivate Russian-style dysfunction in Britain? The answers radiate out from a single word – trust.

Trust is the stuff that binds citizens to each other and their political institutions. It is what allows strangers to believe that they have interests in common as part of a shared political enterprise, and that their elected representatives seek office with the collective interest somewhere in mind. It is what brings people to polling stations in the confidence that they are not Potemkin villages.

Patterns of democracy can be present in a climate of degraded trust, but they are decorative. In Russia, the degra-dation began decades before the USSR unravelled. The Com-munist Party oversaw elections, of a sort. The Soviet constitution of 1936, introduced at the height of Stalin's terror, guaranteed freedom of speech. Everyone still knew that the potential penalty for speaking out was a 3 a.m. knock at the door and a bullet in the neck.

The official line, that socialism was a force for collective emancipation (and offered a higher plane of freedom than bourgeois democracy), was still being parroted in the seventies and eighties, through the stagnant dusk of Soviet senescence. The result was that politics became a ritualized hypocrisy. Everyone understood the sorts of things that had to be said to climb the apparatus of the party, and also that those things were refuted by the facts of Soviet life. A clear distinction emerged between a formalized 'truth' as it had to be expressed in public, and actual truth as it was discussed privately, among trusted friends, as jokes and ironic asides in the realm of inner emigration.

The democratic reforms of the early nineties failed to address that psychological malaise. The connective tissue that might have linked ordinary people to centres of power was not repaired. The form of politics changed; the constitution was rewritten, but soon enough democracy came to be seen as just another doctrine – a new party line extolling new virtues for embroidering onto banners and celebrating at marches, while in reality the same old games continued, played by familiar rules, arbitrated by the same red-faced men, only now they wore imported Italian suits.

In Russia, the absence of trust meant the machinery of democracy was installed on soggy foundations. The equipment was poorly maintained, then vandalized. In Britain, the apparatus has been ticking over for longer, but that doesn't make it indestructible or safe from neglect. There is a slower, more subtle kind of corrosion that degrades long-established institutions.

The telltale symptom is a conviction that anyone who has made it to a certain level of success in public life must be crooked, or mad; that statements of principle are for display only – the kind of thing a politician is meant to say, not expressions of belief. Endemic mistrust hollows politics out until every statement is presumed to be a cynical deception. There is always some theatricality in politics, but democracy itself should not be seen as pure artifice, with real power operating out of sight, in the wings.

Scepticism about politics is not unhealthy in itself. It is logical to doubt the solidity of promises when they are broken so often. Trust should be conditional. A rational sceptic holds out for evidence that a politician is worth following but remains open to persuasion. Sceptics do not automatically reject every statement on the assumption that it exists to hide a nefarious agenda. That is cynicism – the condition of presuming the worst underlying motive of anyone involved in public life.

Then there is a further stage – hypercynicism. It is the state of jaundiced, nihilistic contempt for politics that passes all the way through scepticism and cynicism, full circle back into a kind of credulity. The hypercynic takes the conviction that politics is a sham as reason to get behind strongmen, showmen, despots and fraudsters because they make the performance and deception explicit. Everyone knows they are lying, but the blatancy of the lie – the naked chutzpah of it – wears a defiance that feels like honesty. Or rather, *authenticity* – not pretending to be better than a pretender.

Hypercynicism creates a powerful bond between leader and follower that transcends the requirement for evidence. Hypercynical candidates can't disappoint their supporters because they aren't promising to be truthful. They are admitting that it's all a performance and offering fans the privilege of being part of the show.

(iii) The water and the whale

When you grow up in a country that chooses its government peacefully, it is easy to think of democracy as something that happens in episodes.

There is a campaign, a vote, maybe one party is evicted from power and another one installed. Between those set pieces, life for the vast majority is unpolitical. Some people are drawn to participate more fully than others, perhaps out of a sense of civic duty, or passion for a cause, or the thrill of getting closer to power. Most don't bother.

In a healthy democracy, tuning out from politics needn't imply contempt or disillusionment. It can be an act of trust. It defers judgement to people who care more, outsourcing engagement to activists and obsessives. The unspoken assumption is that the engaged minority broadly represent the whole society and won't wreck everything for the majority

To be an episodic democrat is to have faith in the civic culture of the nation. You don't have to wear confidence in the system as a badge of identity. You don't need to *demand* democracy, because democracy is freely available.

Each election comes along like a whale breaching the surface of the ocean, causing a great splash and spray before plunging back down out of sight. It is memorable, noticeable, but not what the whale is doing most of the time. Between journeys to the surface, it subsists on plankton. If all you care about is the whale, it is easy not to notice incremental changes in water temperature and levels of pollution that might be endangering the ecosystem.

An episodic democrat might be mistrustful of politicians but not hypercynical. There is a presumption that even a government you don't like will respect your rights. There are unspoken parameters that mean one government might be preferable to another, but none will be monstrous. That confidence (or complacency) is a licence to disengage. What's the worst that could happen? Apathy is not a symptom of despair.

For most of my life, most British people have been in that category. I had read about authoritarian governments and knew (or thought I knew) the history that proved democracy to be the most successful principle that humanity had yet found for organizing itself into societies.

Having grown up in the West during the Cold War (I was fifteen when the Berlin Wall came down), I had also come to think of democracy as an automatic aspiration in people who didn't have it. The case against any other system seemed so overwhelming that the only reason *not* to identify as a democrat would be if a bullying government made the public display of it dangerous. This too was a presumption I had to adjust after spending time in Russia.

Nostalgia for the Soviet Union kicked in almost as soon as the Communist Party was out. It was strongest and quickest to take hold in the older generations. They were bankrupted by currency devaluations, lost their pensions, had fewer new avenues for earning and felt more physically vulnerable to lawlessness. But pretty much everyone remembered something fondly from the USSR. Fondness was the seed of future resentment. The application of Western economic ideas imported from countries that had so recently been the enemy came to feel less like liberation, more like occupation.

As Stephen Holmes and Ivan Krastev have written in *The Light That Failed*, the West failed to grasp the vital distinction between Russian eagerness to be rid of a dictatorial Communist Party and resilient attachment to the Soviet Union as a *country*, including the territories that broke away to form independent states. The USSR had been a motherland. Its dismemberment was disorienting and humiliating.

I argued about this often with my Russian friends. I tried to explain how the anarchic swindle they were calling democracy was not a fair representation of the real thing. One common response was that Russia was too vast and its people too unruly or too steeped in religious traditions of collective submission to be governed by anything other than the iron will of a strongman.

Just as often, I was rebuked for my naivety in thinking that democracy was real in other countries. It was a sham everywhere, I was told. Surely I must know that elections always followed a script written by power-brokers and puppet-masters behind the scenes. When people learned that I was a journalist, they pitied me for trying to get to the bottom of Russian politics or laughed at me for thinking there was a bottom to reach. At the end of every story was a tunnel leading to a secret chamber that joined a mysterious passageway, at the end of which was a locked door, behind which was a winding stairwell that connected to a whole new labyrinth.

The idea that the media might report events truthfully was alien. Everyone had an agenda, I was told. And a price. The truth was set by the highest bidder. There was not much distinction between political analysis and conspiracy theory. Both had their origin in the same analytic maxim: there was power and there was you. Your options were to submit to the power or find a way to make it work on your behalf: pay a bribe, lever some old contact, do a deal and carve out whatever portion of influence you could muster to provide for yourself and your family.

The idea that a politician might feel some democratic vocation to represent your needs was ludicrous; childish. The claim that such politicians existed in Britain was given short shrift. Maybe the sham was more sophisticated in the West, I was told. Maybe the rules were more elaborate and the costumes better designed, but the play was the same.

Putin was shrewd in weaponizing popular resentment that had built against Western models of government. He did not immediately reject democracy, human rights, pluralism and rule of law, but gradually subverted and diminished them. He did not reform gangster capitalism. He harnessed it to the last remaining functional part of Soviet bureaucracy – the security services that had given him his professional start in life. Then he fuelled the whole enterprise with militant national revivalism. Larceny on a massive scale was still permitted as long as it paid tribute to the new boss in the Kremlin.

Putin's steely sobriety made a refreshing enough change from the drunken, flabby anarchy of the Boris Yeltsin years that he could have won elections without cheating. But he didn't take any chances. Faking elections is about much more than the mechanics of stitching up power. Looking back to that empty polling station in Grozny, the bunting, the bored election officials and the overwhelming victory conjured from empty ballot boxes, what stands out is the brazenness of it, verging on absurdity.

We were not fooled, but we were not supposed to be fooled. The trip was only superficially meant to show democracy in action. At the time, I imagined the spectacle was put on for the press in the hope of getting favourable reviews. But seeing it from that angle misunderstood the function of electoral fraud. Putin did not want approval from us any more than he expected his own voters to be taken in by a charade of con-sultation. The Potemkin election is caricature, not counterfeit. It is not fakery that is designed to be passed off as the genuine article, but a pastiche.

The artifice is explicit because flagrant cheating and getting away with it is a way of asserting power. It sends a signal to the population that the apparatus of democracy can be put up and pulled down on a whim; that the state's control exists on a higher plane – untouchable. As journalists in Chechnya, we weren't the audience for the pantomime, we were props on stage.

The Potemkin election is part of a process of inducing a deeper Potemkin *syndrome* in a society, characterized by a view that the only reason anyone would get involved in politics in the first place is to be part of the deception. In a country afflicted by Potemkin syndrome, the way to feel empowered is to surrender to powerlessness; to be so sincere in your cheers for the liars that the lies start to feel true.

Holmes and Krastev have described Putin's methods as a 'violent parody' of Western styles, sending up democracy by doing it badly at home but also subverting it abroad. That is what interference in the 2016 US presidential ballot was all about. It suited the Kremlin to have Trump elected president, since that would strategically weaken the old superpower adversary. But just as important, or more so, it suited Putin to have US politics consumed with arguments about the legitimacy of an election. It didn't really matter who won, as long as there was recognition that meddlesome spooky Russian provocateurs might have skewed the result.

When American elections take a darkly farcical turn, it confirms the idea that democracy itself is a charade and only suckers take it at face value. The parody advances the view that representative government is a fairy tale for fools and hypocrites. The smart people see through it. For ordinary citizens, the reward for that insight is world-weary satisfaction at being in on the scam. There is a depth of suspicion that provides a kind of bleak insulation against false hope. The hypercynical society, padded with a fatalistic presumption that nothing will get better, is not spurred to revolt by the stab of disappointment.

I left Russia in 2003, tired, hungover, eager to get back to a country where it wasn't preposterous to describe MPs as public servants and where journalism didn't always feel like the losing side in a war of attrition against fact-based reality. I knew that British politicians were capable of corruption and deception, but I liked the idea of doing my job in a political system that still recognized a realm of truth independent of what the regime decreed it to be. I had seen how a democracy became parched and shrivelled without the irrigation of trust. I had watched one die. I took comfort in the thought that nothing of the sort could happen back home.

CHAPTER 6

FRACKING DEMOCRACY

A mixture of gullibility and cynicism had been an outstanding characteristic of mob mentality before it became an everyday phenomenon of masses. In an ever-changing, incomprehensible world the masses had reached the point where they would, at the same time, believe everything and nothing, think that everything *is* possible and that nothing was true. The mixture in itself was remarkable enough, because it spelled the end of the illusion that gullibility was a weakness of unsuspecting primitive souls and cynicism the vice of superior and refined minds. Mass propaganda discovered that its audience was ready at all times to believe the worst, no matter how absurd, and did not particularly object to being deceived because it held every statement to be a lie anyhow.

Hannah Arendt

(i) Flooding the zone

In March 2018, Vladimir Putin started a fourth term as Russia's president.* British politics was bogged down deep in trench

---

* He had also served a term as prime minister, wielding presidential powers, as a ruse to get around a constitutional prohibition on any one candidate taking more than two consecutive terms. He has since ironed that wrinkle out of the constitution.

warfare over Brexit. I was depressed about the state we were in; alarmed by the ominous groaning and creaking that sounded like foundations giving way beneath our once stable parliamentary democracy. I had been back from Moscow for a while, but stayed in touch with old friends. Occasionally, we would speak on the phone, and they would remind me how lucky I was to still be shocked by the state of politics. The emotion testified to a residual belief that a higher standard of leadership was available. I remember one such conversation with my friend Dmitri, a few days after Putin had won his election with 78 per cent of the vote.

Dmitri is an Anglophile in every respect, as sure of British democratic resilience as he is persuaded by the culinary genius of Marmite. He listened patiently as I recounted my frustrations with Westminster, my conviction that Brexit was a monstrous folly. He cut me short when I started describing the dismay of Remainers the morning after the referendum when they learned how many of their compatriots had voted for national ruin: 'Listen, Raf, I'm sure it was hard for those people that morning. But at least they got to go to bed the night before not yet knowing what the result would be.'

I often recall that comment as a corrective to the miserable view that every misstep in British politics is hastening us towards tyranny; as if there is only one way that governments go bad and no coming back once they start down that path.

There are many different flavours of maladministration short of dictatorship, from mildly incompetent to rampantly corrupt. As long as the outcomes of our elections are unpredictable, we can at least take comfort in the prospect of today's hapless rulers becoming tomorrow's ineffectual opposition.

Dmitri's rebuke came at a time when I was feeling demoralized by politics in a particular way – a feeling unnervingly reminiscent of my time in Moscow. It is hard to characterize exactly. I can pinpoint the moment I made the connection because the way it struck me was almost physical, the way a distinctive smell can transport you back to a specific place and time. I was walking down Victoria Street towards the Palace of Westminster, fretting over some inanity that was occupying the morning's headlines, when I was overwhelmed by déjà vu.

But it wasn't a vague sense of the scene being familiar. It was a visceral, almost hallucinatory transportation back to a different time in my career, so strong that it stopped me in my tracks. Something about British politics *tasted Russian*.

To be clear, I didn't think that Britain was about to slump into Putin-style authoritarianism. I don't think it is now. The likeness was recognizable but intangible, which is why I compare it to a taste, or maybe a smell. It was something about the flavour of arguments, their caustic bite; something in the way people were being denounced not for the content of their arguments but for the sinister motive presumed to lie beneath the surface; something in the presumption of bad faith in every rival stance; the whiff of hypercynicism.

Needless to say, much of what I am describing was expressed online. I don't claim to have some sixth sense that could sniff out digital saboteurs sent by the Kremlin to meddle with our elections. Britain didn't need help from Russian security services to polarize itself and foment bitterness on the internet. But that help was there.

Russia's Internet Research Agency has been operating from the Olgino district of St Petersburg since 2013, although the state had been monitoring and disrupting digital debate long before that. (Even a decade earlier, when I wrote something about Russia's HIV crisis, I was met with a barrage of nearly identical online comments denouncing my report as Western propaganda covering up a NATO plot to use AIDS as a weapon.)

The Olgino Trolls, as they are sometimes known in Russia, spread misinformation and slander to discredit domestic opposition and promote Kremlin agendas abroad. In any country where there is an election or crisis of interest to Moscow, the troll armies get to work taking sides, sowing discord, trampling dirt into the pool of facts to muddy the waters. When there is a terrorist attack, the bot accounts are first to fabricate false leads and share the most hysterical, bigoted takes on social media. By some estimates, anywhere between a third and two thirds of all web traffic is automated bot accounts. A lot of that is non-political junk, but even if a fraction of it is malicious provocation, there will be a non-negligible effect on the tone of public discourse.

It isn't just the Russians. China, Iran and North Korea are in on the act too, but the method was pioneered by the Kremlin. The strategy has been dubbed 'managed chaos'. Russia's financial debilitation after the Cold War changed the character of the rivalry with the US and European countries. Efforts at partnership failed, not least because Moscow could not accept the junior status imposed by its shrunken economy. So a new form of insidious confrontation was developed. As a 2018 paper for the Center for European Policy Analysis, a Washington-based think tank, put it: 'The "chaos strategy" calculates that a relatively weakened Kremlin can avoid direct competition with the West to still successfully compete by splintering its opponents' alliances, dividing them internally, and undermining their political systems.'

To that end, it is clear why Kremlin agents took an interest in helping Donald Trump reach the White House, and also why they meddled in matters like Scottish independence and Brexit. How effective they are is hard to quantify. To imagine that troll states have hoodwinked whole electorates is paranoid; pretending there was no impact is naive.

Brexit enthusiasts were reluctant to admit that Putin was clapping along to their tune (and financing their pipers). They had even more reason to be coy after the invasion of Ukraine, when it became unfashionable for Western nationalists to be openly impressed by Putin. Nigel Farage once claimed to admire the Russian president 'as an operator'.

British Eurosceptics sang harmony to a Kremlin melody on the annexation of Crimea in 2014. Always on the lookout for reasons to despise Brussels, Britain's anti-EU politicians embraced the Putinist view that Europe had provoked the crisis by doing trade deals with the government in Kyiv. Farage accused the EU of running a 'militarist and expansionist' foreign policy.* In 2016, Boris Johnson told a referendum rally that the EU's trade partnership agreement with Ukraine had 'caused real trouble' and that things 'went wrong' there because 'all the EU can do in this question is cause confusion'. Putin no doubt agreed.

---

* Farage's entourage also had private contact with the Putin regime. His friend and financier Arron Banks enjoyed a long, vodka-drenched lunch with the Russian ambassador to Britain in November 2015. The introduction had been made by someone Banks described as 'a shady character called Oleg' who had attended a UKIP conference in Doncaster. 'Oleg' was, in fact, Alexander Udod, a member of the Russian intelligence service who would later be expelled from the UK.

Whether Kremlin subterfuge tipped the scales for Brexit is unknowable. Remainers exaggerate the impact to avoid conceding how thoroughly they lost a domestic argument.* It is more fruitful to consider how the interference is meant to work. What is the vulnerability being exploited?

Russia sows discord around divisive causes because polarized societies are harder to govern.† In Britain, the most fruitful targets have been constitutional questions that resist management through the channels of representative democracy – Brexit and Scottish independence. Why else would Alex Salmond, former leader of the Scottish National Party and first minister of Scotland, have been given his own talk show on *RT*, the international channel of Kremlin propaganda? (For the same reason, Kremlin troll armies swarm all over the digital front line of Catalonia's demands for independence from Spain.)

It doesn't really matter which side wins as long as everyone is more embittered and opinion is more entrenched by the process. The primary goal is to aggravate grievance, spread doubt about the veracity of all sources and trigger a chain reaction of radicalization. It is a malicious pollution of the information space that makes it hard to evaluate what is true, inviting the hypercynical conclusion that truth itself is unavailable from the established political channels. The result is shrunken bandwidth for moderation and compromise,

---

* The same is true with the US presidential election in 2016, where Russian meddling was egregious and beyond doubt. A conviction that victory was stolen from Hillary Clinton did not help Democrats come to terms with the deeper causes of support for Donald Trump, which was organic to the soil of American culture and not simply cooked up in a secret Russian laboratory.

† For the same reason, the Kremlin has channelled money into the coffers of political parties in various Western democracies.

which limits the capacity of government to balance rival social interests.

Wherever a culture war burns, malignant online actors spray petrol on the flames. A US Senate committee investigation found that Russian-based accounts were responsible for posting in one corner of the internet images celebrating the Confederate flag, and in another, messages in support of the Black Lives Matter campaign. An internal Facebook report, leaked to the *MIT Technology Review* in September 2021, found that the social media giant's most viewed content for Christian and African-American users during the 2020 presidential election had been generated by Eastern European troll farms. Those pages were part of a network that had reached the eyeballs of nearly half of all Americans.

The US was the biggest target, but Britain was also in the line of fire. The scale of these operations has grown in recent years, but they were up and running before many users were even aware that bots and fake news were a thing. How significant their impact is is hard to know. In 2020, Alex Younger, former head of MI6, made a rare public intervention on this subject. In an interview with the *Financial Times*, he identified two common mistakes in response to Russian meddling:

> The first is to do Russia's job for them by bigging it up; I haven't seen in the UK any occasion where this stuff has made a strategic difference. Secondly, and related, I think we should keep this in proportion. The Russians did not create the things that divide us – we did that. They are adept, albeit in a rather crass manner, at exacerbating those things and I believe that we should prevent that.

That second point is vital. Misinformation and provocation work by punching bruises that we land on each other. They work as techniques for sabotaging democracy by inflating prejudice on either side of a divide to the point where common language is impossible. The purpose is to escalate mutual mistrust so that rival social factions stop seeing each other as civil adversaries within a unified political system and start despising each other as unspeakably wrong; not competitors, but enemies; not advocates for legitimate alternative policy but evildoers.

That is a sabotage of the basic function of representative democracy. It negates the idea that different interest groups can all be accommodated under one system as long as they accept only partial satisfaction of their demands.

As a method of political engineering, it is analogous to fracking for shale gas. That process involves drilling down into rock and pumping in fluid to create splits and fissures, breaking subterranean structures to release trapped hydrocarbon stores. When fracking a democracy, the same principle applies. You drill in places where there is a reservoir of combustible fury buried beneath sediments of democratic consensus. If you pump enough partisan argument, polemic, emotive imagery and fake news into the cultural substrata, the encasing rock fractures. The flammable gas is released. Domestic politicians go along with that process, wittingly or not, because there is so much energy in those wells.

Fracking democracy releases the fuel for hypercynical campaigns. It spreads the impression that nothing in the media can be believed, everyone is lying, and the only truth that matters is found in devotion to your candidate. Or, as Steve

Bannon, Donald Trump's former campaign strategist, said in 2018: 'The real opposition is the media. And the way to deal with them is to flood the zone with shit.'

The winning side in an election in the West will never admit to complicity with a Kremlin agenda, but every populist campaign pollutes the water and fouls the political air to the benefit of authoritarians everywhere. The technique of winning power by wilfully inflaming social division is an aggression against the idea that citizens with opposing views might still find a common purpose in democracy.

(ii) Is everything sacred?

To be clear: the fracking of British democracy is not something that is perpetrated against the country by foreign agents. It is something we do to ourselves, with mischievous outsiders as marginal accomplices.

A fracked political system is marked by mistrust on two axes – the horizontal one between citizens and the vertical between institutions of government and the people being governed. It will be polarized also in two dimensions. Polarization can describe a clustering of opinion around remote ends of a left–right spectrum (or at poles of liberal and authoritarian opinion). That in itself needn't be socially calamitous. People can hold vastly divergent views and still get along. The more pungent effect is what social scientists call 'affective polarization' – finding opposite views emotionally rebarbative; not wanting to spend time with someone who thinks differently on a hot-button topic; not wanting one's children to marry someone from a different political tribe.

Opinion polls suggest Britain is going down that path. A survey of the public mood by the Policy Institute at King's College London found very high levels of mutual distrust and misunderstanding between voters in the December 2019 general election. Asked to describe how warmly or coldly they were disposed to the other side on a 'feeling thermometer', Labour supporters ranked Tories at a chilly 15 out of 100; Tories felt a fraction warmer, 18, when thinking about Labour people.* By way of comparison, Democrats and Republicans in the 2016 US presidential election – notoriously unharmonious – felt respectively 29 and 31 degrees of warmth to each other.

An opinion poll from 2017 found that only around half of Labour and Conservative voters were happy to talk to someone of the opposing affiliation. Around a quarter of Conservatives were relaxed about the idea of their child marrying a Labour voter. Labour supporters were more tribal still, with only a fifth saying they could tolerate their progeny being betrothed to a Tory. (The divides were similar between Brexit supporters and Remainers.)

As for trust in government and the political system more generally, the evidence suggests decline. A 2021 survey found that just under two thirds of respondents agreed with the statement that democracy was 'rigged to serve the rich and influential'. Another poll in the same year found 63 per cent believing politicians were 'merely out for themselves'. The other options were motivation by party interest and service to the

---

* Although the coldest temperature recorded of all was Tory voters' feelings about Jeremy Corbyn – a freezing 3 degrees.

country at large. The equivalent figure when the same question was asked in 2014 was 48 per cent. When it was first asked in 1944, the number was 35 per cent.

In July 2022, in a survey of 10,000 people for Tortoise Media which asked respondents whether they thought the British political system was democratic, 34 per cent said it was not. The British Social Attitudes survey notes a general decline over the past generation in the number of people believing politicians serve any kind of higher national purpose.

A particularly worrying sign is high numbers of young people thinking democracy doesn't work. Research in September 2022 by Onward, a moderate Conservative think tank, looked at the share of people aged 18–34 supporting the idea of 'a strong leader who does not have to worry about parliament or elections'. Backing for that proposition was 60 per cent, double what it had been 20 years previously. Nearly half of the same cohort believed that 'military rule would be a good way to run the country'. In 1999, that had been 9 per cent.

The British Election Survey finds a generational decline in respondents' likelihood to agree with the statement that 'it's everyone's duty to vote.' In 1987, 76 per cent felt that way. That had dropped to 62 per cent by 2011, when the question was last asked. But the same surveys find *interest* in politics to be steady or rising over the same period.

Some forms of participation – writing to MPs and signing petitions – have become more prolific. That might reflect the increased ease of firing off an email or putting a name into a website compared to the old analogue ways of passing on an opinion, but a fully despondent population wouldn't bother even clicking send on an e-petition.

It isn't clear what that increase in attention to politics says about the temper of engagement. A society in which rival clans of prolific petition-signers lobby their MPs and shout at each other on the internet might also contain a large number of people who feel alienated by the rancorous tone of debate.

The person who sends a hundred hand-written letters to politicians and journalists, urging them do something about the Illuminati plot to enslave humanity – and I periodically get these letters – is a lot more engaged than someone who sends none. That isn't a barometer of democratic well-being.

Opinion polls suggest that conspiratorial thinking is rampant. A 2018 survey found 44 per cent of people agreeing with the statement: 'even though we live in what's called a democracy, a few people will always run things in this country anyway.' In a comparative poll of different national views from 2021, 28 per cent of British respondents thought it was either definitely true or probably true that 'regardless of who is officially in charge of governments and other organizations, there is a single group of people who secretly control events and rule the world together.' It should be added that those numbers are not especially high by international standards. When asked the same question, more than a third of Americans bought the idea of a secret single world government.*

It is hard to be precise about the role of the internet in those trends. Polarization and mistrust are not discoveries of the digital age. What does appear to be changing under technological

---

* Top of the suspicion league on that question was Nigeria – 78 per cent. South Africa wasn't far behind. Generally there looks to be a correlation between the dysfunction of democratic practice, corruption and popular faith in conspiracy theory.

influence is the character of politics. There have always been people with opposing views who prefer like-minded company and people who think the government is full of crooks. But social media appears to be evangelizing for that view and turning it implacable. It is a vast engine of radicalization.

The architecture and algorithms of social media accelerate innate tendencies to prejudice and a natural inclination to reject unwelcome evidence. We select followers and sift for data that confirm what we want to believe is true. The human mind has evolved to prioritize emotive confirmation of what *feels* right over dispassionate evaluation of what is in fact the case.

Through Facebook, Twitter, Instagram, TikTok we furnish cosy information silos for ourselves. They are not impermeable. Dissenting views get through, but they will be presented to us in terms that invite ridicule or scorn, as exemplars of wrong thinking that invite a withdrawal of empathy from anyone foolish enough to hold such a dumb opinion in good faith.

That would not be a problem if we wore our political prejudices lightly and were able to separate them from broader social judgements about our neighbours. But radicalization works by fusing opinions and identity. It is the fusion of judgement about public policy – which candidate to support; whether taxes should go up or down – to more intimate feelings about identity and morality – who is a good person; what is a threat to ourselves and our community.*

It is hard to dislodge or revise an opinion that defines our feelings of belonging to a group. How we view the relative

---

* This shift can even be traced in magnetic resonance imagery of the brain, where expression of radically felt views and more rationally considered ones illuminate different cerebral regions.

merits of our football club, for example, will have a different intensity to how we judge the superiority of one cereal brand to another. Some political views are the anchor for our sense of how the world is morally constructed, and how we fit into it. In psychological terms, those are the views we hold *sacred*.

Everyone has sacred beliefs, although we might not recognize them as such, especially if they are not obviously connected to spiritual or religious practice. Sacred beliefs, as recognized by modern psychology,* do not have to be attached to deities or supernatural forces. They are the beliefs that have been cemented into the edifice of selfhood.

Someone might vote Labour, for example, because on balance they prefer the look of the party leader or a particular policy. That is a loose allegiance. For the person who wears a T-shirt with the slogan 'Never Kissed a Tory', Labour is not a secular political choice any more. It is sacred.

The cohesion of our identity is destabilized if the truth of our sacred values is undermined, which is why people work hard – consciously and subconsciously – to resist any challenge to them. Once a view becomes sacred, the existence of valid alternatives is discounted.

Social media has a way of intensifying views into that zone where dissent is perceived as existential threat. It *sacralizes* politics. The passion with which we care about things becomes more ardent. The social cost of changing our minds or moderating our views gets inflated. When the information

---

* It has been argued by Jonathan Haidt, Drew Westen and others that conservatives are generally better at recognizing and targeting the potency of sacred values in the formation of political opinion and so are more effective in election campaigns.

space we inhabit has been tailored to fit our prejudices and reinforce our identities, we find it harder to discard opinions that we might once have carried more lightly.

This isn't something unique to the internet. Social pressures have always policed boundaries of opinion. If your weekends are spent hunting and fishing with your best friends, you have powerful motives not to dwell on the arguments for vegetarianism. We are social animals. It is rational to prefer comfortable agreement with the people around you to contrarian solitude.

But the dynamic is accelerated online, where lines of partisanship are enforced by mobs that dispense with the niceties of analogue social conduct. The penalty for saying the wrong thing can be merciless and relentless. No one who has been at the bottom of an internet pile-on is in a hurry to repeat the experience.

Radicalization and polarization reinforce each other in a feedback loop. The problem is not necessarily an unbridgeable distance between opinions but the ferocity of emotion that is excited by contact with a different view. Bridging the gap (or scaling the high walls between positions that are closer than they seem) is a task requiring calm, reflective thought. Unfortunately, too, it is made harder by digital platforms that have a commercial incentive to keep us skittish and angry.

(iii) Attention deficit democracy

There is no single ideology encoded in the internet, but it favours certain modes of political expression. It is biased in favour of bias. The business model of social media depends on impulsive behaviour at the expense of rational reflection. Most of the services we use online are ostensibly free. Google doesn't charge for search results. It costs nothing to open a Facebook account. The real transaction is a trade in the data we supply every time we search, comment, share, like, sell, buy, ask a question of Amazon's Alexa, post or rate anything.

With every click (or step we take with our phone's location accessible by satellite monitoring), we are communicating preferences that help the companies build predictive models of human behaviour that become targeted ads and customized services. The machine learns our tastes and anticipates our needs. If your Facebook profile is steeped in chatter about golf, an online golfing paraphernalia store will pay for access to your eyeballs. The same mechanism generates a precious trove of data to anyone wanting to organize a political campaign. Your prejudices can be fed back to you as tailor-made messages from the candidate.*

We make better customers when we communicate those tastes with minimal consideration. An algorithm that wants to sell us stuff learns most about our needs when we indulge them on impulse. The most lucrative customer for Facebook is one who spends a lot of unthinking time on the network. Social media platforms are designed to hook us in and inhibit the methodical (and frugal) thinking that might overrule a spontaneous purchase. Hooked is the word, because the experience is addictive.

---

* This is not inherently wicked or new, it should be noted. Politicians have always said what they think their audience wants to hear. The greater concern from the point of view of democratic accountability is what permissions are granted for the use of personal data and who is paying for online campaigns – an issue on which UK election law is hopelessly out of date.

Tristan Harris, a former Google designer, has described the smartphone as 'the slot machine in your pocket' because of the way it pays out doses of reward to a template more commonly associated with gambling addiction. The pattern of notifications – intermittent and of varying value – provokes the brain into checking each time in the hope of hitting a jackpot.

The same principle applies in video games, where points and treasures are distributed on a schedule that is neither regular enough to be predictable nor rare enough that the player quits. Sean Parker, a former president of Facebook, described the calculation explicitly in a 2017 interview:

> The thought process was all about, 'How do we consume as much of your time and conscious attention as possible? And that means that we need to sort of give you a little dopamine hit every once in a while, because someone liked or commented on a photo or a post or whatever, and that's going to get you to contribute more content, and that's going to get you more likes and comments. It's a social validation feedback loop . . . You're exploiting a vulnerability in human psychology.

The game is designed to keep us playing, and on social media, life is gamified. It is a race to acquire friends and Twitter followers, likes and retweets. From the companies' perspective, those are the currencies that keep you on the platform for longer. The commodity is attention, and it doesn't really matter whether it was a cat picture, a football score or an anti-vaccine video that induced the click. It makes no difference whether or not the content in an article is true.

The concept of an 'attention economy' was coined before the internet wrote it into the business model of a multi-trillion-dollar industry. It was first theorized in the 1970s by computer scientist and psychologist (and Nobel laureate) Herbert A. Simon. As he put it:

> In an information-rich world, the wealth of information means a dearth of something else: a scarcity of whatever it is that information consumes. What information consumes is rather obvious: it consumes the attention of its recipients. Hence a wealth of information creates a poverty of attention.

The more crowded the information marketplace, the harder it is for bland facts to compete with more lurid fare. Palates that are jaded need higher doses of spice. In politics, that creates incentives to wilful provocation. One way to catch the attention of a large audience is to stir a smaller one into a lather of indignation. In politics, infuriating the other side can be an effective campaign technique to amplify a core message.

An infamous case in recent political memory was the dishonest claim painted on the side of a Vote Leave battle bus: 'We send the EU £350 million a week. Let's fund our NHS instead.' Remainers were incensed by the £350 million number, which had no meaningful basis in fact. But attacks on that figure still served the underlying Brexit goal, which was to implant in voters' minds an idea: EU membership cost a load of money – it didn't really matter how much.

For social media platforms and publishers, extreme opinions are doubly lucrative, shared once by those who passionately agree and then again by the other side as exemplars of wrongness.

The arena where political news and ideas are shared is sustained in emotional frenzy, which is not the mental state conducive to judicious moderation. The information machinery bypasses those parts of our cognition – the dispassionate, ruminative cerebral functions – that deal with impulse control and regulate fight-or-flight, adrenaline-fuelled reaction.

Some of the most sophisticated technologies developed by our species have been made subordinate to the primitive side of our nature. Then we wired that machinery up to the heart of democracy. Repetitive troglodyte clicking is a feature, not a bug, in the system of politics online.

There is a connection between the way internet commerce is set up to short-circuit rational judgement, and the political effectiveness of populist and nationalist candidates. The common appeal is immediacy. One-click consumer culture is the enemy of deferred gratification. Whatever the problem, the solution is here and now. This is analogous to the impatience that demagogues exploit when campaigning against the frustrations of representative democracy.

Every second of the political day on social media is a referendum on whatever feels most urgent in the moment. The high frequency of that cycle makes it harder to distinguish between what is noisy and what is important. It militates against the debate of priorities, which is part of the negotiation of trade-offs necessary for pluralist politics to function. The algorithms and troglodyte impulses that make us eager buyers of trash we don't need also stoke our appetite for junk politics.

The effect is infantilizing, in the sense that it infuses politics with a toddlerish temperament – wanting things right now;

having tantrums when they are denied. (Chris Wetherell, the software developer who created the retweet function for Twitter, worried about exactly this bypass of adult cognition when he reflected that 'we might have just handed a four-year-old a loaded weapon.')

It isn't that Facebook, Twitter or any other tech company set out with the goal of corrupting democracy. The embitterment of debate and shrinkage of neutral spaces where compromise might be available just happen to be the commercial imperative – the online bazaar is also a public square. The trading platform is also a service that disables critical judgement in politics.

The damage goes deeper than surface disputes that divide public opinion. It is a structural assault on the bedrock of collective belonging to a single political community. It unpicks the conceptual basis of what we call, as a singular noun, 'the public', as distinct from a multitude of querulous individuals or tribes. It is hard to have a debate about the best course of action when the information space has been segregated into comfort zones, each with its own protective barricade against distressing counter-argument.

In such a disaggregated post-public realm, it is hard to agree on what matters, and hard even to settle on a standard account of what constitutes reality – whether the crowd at a presidential inauguration was big or small; whether or not COVID is real.

Scientifically demonstrable facts have not been eliminated from public life, as the common 'post-truth' lament would imply. COVID was killing people whether they believed in it or not. Pandemic policy in Britain might not have been a prompt or exact enactment of what government scientists recommended,* but nor did it go chasing after bizarre superstitions.

The more subtle and pernicious aspect of post-truth media is the amount of energy that ends up being consumed in the competition to define basic facts that shouldn't even need contesting. That accelerates the fracking of democracy and the corrosion of trust in civil institutions. It aggravates the Potemkin syndrome.

A vicious cycle begins. The overwhelming complexity of modern life is made more alarming by the digital frenzy, which in turn stimulates an appetite for comforting fictions about the world. We use selective information tools to insulate ourselves from spiky truths. In those conditions, voters are attracted to candidates who reflect their fear and anger back at them, validating their sense of grievance and offering the solace of simple solutions.

But those candidates are hopelessly ill-equipped to handle the actual challenges of government. Once elected, they fail to deliver the gratification that was promised. Then begins the hunt for scapegoats. Frustration and anger with the political system becomes both cause and effect of political fury. Staggering through that red mist, we lose sight of what we have in common.

(iv) Us and them

Jo Cox had been in Parliament for just over a year before her assassination. Her maiden speech in the House of Commons was a celebration of cultural diversity in her constituency, Batley

---

* More on this in later chapters. Science and politics will always have an uneasy relationship, because the dictates of political ambition so often contradict evidence that a specific policy is failing.

and Spen. The peroration became her epitaph: 'We are far more united and have far more in common than that which divides us.' That is usually true. More important, perhaps, it is something that most people want to believe, which is the necessary foundation for it becoming true.

The appetite for solidarity was displayed every Thursday evening during the pandemic, when we stood on our doorsteps and clapped in tribute to health workers. Confinement increased our craving for contact. We waved to neighbours we had somehow failed to meet in all the years before social distance was mandated by public health regulations. We felt closer because intimacy was forbidden. That spirit had dissipated even before the regulations were lifted. The polarizing dynamics of British politics, made all the more vigorous by a divisive prime minister, overwhelmed the cohesive urge of the public.

On 15 October 2021, another MP was murdered. Sir David Amess, the Conservative MP for Southend West, was stabbed in his constituency. The attacker, Ali Harbi Ali, was a freelance affiliate of the Islamic State jihadist group in Syria. Like Cox's assassin, Ali had radicalized himself in isolation.

Britain likes to think of itself as a country where politics is conducted within commonly understood civil parameters. There is supposed to be a mainstream zone densely populated with democrats, beyond which lies a fringe where nutters dwell (some harmless, some violent). There is no fixed boundary in reality. The delineation of moderate and extreme is always in motion, but the conception of a line is essential for democratic self-belief. It is one of the ways we recognize that differences of party affiliation are subordinate to the higher value of peaceful, plural politics as a communal property. In the civic zone, there is no need to kill politicians for a cause, because regime change can be effected by voting.

Assassinations force the question of how and why some people reject that view. In the aftermath of David Amess's death, there was a surge of debate about incivility and the coarsening of public discourse. There was cross-party agreement that the tone of politics had become toxic, but no consensus on the causes of decline, or when it had started. There is not always a clear distinction between personal abuse and legitimate opposition, especially when a politician's reprobate character is the reason their policies are failing. Does it demean politics to call a prime minister who tells lies a liar?

People have always disagreed about stuff. There was no golden age of democratic discourse when rival views were debated in every market square with only analytical rigour and no emotional rancour.

When journalists of a certain age complain about the proliferation of falsehood and irresponsible rabble-rousing online, they gloss over the hysterical partisanship that is the normal idiom of the British tabloid newspapers, and is even celebrated as robustness in the free press. When the charlatan Andrew Wakefield had a bogus theory connecting the MMR vaccine to autism, he didn't need Facebook to spread the myth. The *Daily Mail* eagerly took up the cause.

Political abuse was not invented by social media. The Museum of London has a collection of letters sent to prominent suffragettes, containing threats of violence and aggressive misogyny. 'You set of sickening fools,' writes one irate man. 'If you have no homes, no husbands, no children, no relations, why don't you just drown yourselves out of the way?'

Often the collective memory of less embittered times relates to periods of external threat – the Blitz spirit, for example, which might provide a happy metaphor for solidarity, though having the Luftwaffe overhead is hardly a desirable model to copy.

When people fondly recall the good old days, characterized by more genteel debate, they also overlook the role that class deference and hierarchies of race and gender played in that more polite yesteryear. More argumentative politics is partly a function of people who were once excluded from the arguments raising their voices. A society in which a wide range of diverse opinions can freely be expressed is in better democratic health than one in which there is an unquestioned orthodoxy or state-controlled view.

The men who murdered Jo Cox and David Amess were hardly typical of the British voter. The journey from private fulmination to actual violence is rare, and no one knows what other social and pathological factors send someone down that path. The chain of causation that links acts of terror to the wider culture of contempt for politics and hatred of politicians is unproven. It is certainly plausible that decay of civility online has a wider impact, tearing at the threads that weave individuals into a social fabric, normalizing unrestrained aggression. Combine that with the radicalizing function of digital media, and you have a powerful engine for turning a disliked politician into a hated enemy and a hated enemy into an existential menace that must be eliminated with violence.

In the days after Amess's murder, MPs began speaking more openly about the volume of abuse they get online and in the street – death threats, rape threats, racism, misogyny, vandalized offices, intimidated staff. Politicians started saying in public what many journalists had heard them say before in private. Pervasive public hostility was taxing their health and giving them cause to fear for their partners and kids. 'I did try to keep it from them when they were smaller,' Labour's Jess Phillips said in a TV interview. 'But when the police are coming round weekly to take statements, the children start to notice these things.'

Two MPs have been murdered in the past two decades, but there have been near misses too. In 2010, Stephen Timms was stabbed in his East Ham constituency surgery by Roshonara Choudhry, an Islamist radical. In 2019, Jack Renshaw, a neo-Nazi, was jailed for plotting to murder Rosie Cooper, MP for West Lancashire. Renshaw was a member of National Action, a far-right faction that expressed support for Thomas Mair's attack on Jo Cox and was banned under anti-terrorism law in 2016.

Those cases may be few, but there are enough of them to make anyone uneasy at the sight – increasingly common – of angry crowds mobbing MPs as they walk down Whitehall. It seems to have become part of the repertoire of political participation. A gang of irate protesters, or sometimes just a determined individual, sees a prominent public figure going about their business and starts haranguing them. In recent years, videos of these ambushes have circulated online, with Keir Starmer, Michael Gove and Jacob Rees-Mogg on the receiving end of the tirade. In the latter case, the minister was accompanied by his 12-year-old son, who had to witness a stranger bellowing 'Nazi arsehole' at his dad.

What does abuse of politicians convey, beyond loss of temper? A generous interpretation is that it describes broken confidence in conventional democratic channels (an explanation, not an excuse). If the ruling class is deemed remote, unresponsive, unreachable, there is a natural impulse to turn up the volume. People who feel thwarted in life take their frustrations out on the perceived cause of their disempowerment – the politicians who have the power. Abuse is then conceived by the abuser as an act of rebellion. The attackers exonerate themselves from responsibility to behave by codes of conduct designed, as they see it, to uphold a system of oppression.

To think that way takes a Potemkinized view of the relationship between power and the citizen. It is a perception of politicians (and their media lackeys) as 'them' – alien, dedicated to malfeasance – in league against 'us', the ordinary people. Those terms are incompatible with the idea of representative democracy, where MPs are elected from among the people to exercise judgement on their behalf and mediate their interests by proxy. Perhaps the most lethal effect of a fracked democracy is this entrenchment of them-and-us politics when the system can only function on the understanding that they *are* us.

CHAPTER 7

OFF BALANCE

It is reasonable to have perfection in our eye that we may always advance toward it, though we know it can never be reached.

Samuel Johnson

(i) The Fitzgerald problem

If I had known I was going to go viral, I would have ironed my shirt.

It was a crisp, sunny Friday in June and I had been invited to appear as a guest pundit on the BBC's *Daily Politics* programme. The topic was Brexit. Of course. This was 2019; there were no other topics. Towards the end of the show, a question came my way and I disgorged some of the frustration that had been building inside me over the previous half-hour of the show; and the previous four years. The whole of British politics was consumed in debating the European question on terms that bore no relationship to reality, I said. From the outside we looked like a country that had abandoned its belief in gravity. Words to that effect.

I left the studio feeling as I always do after a live broadcast – relieved that I managed not to swear and wishing I had not looked like someone who slept in his clothes. Then the messages started pinging on my phone. Colleagues, family, friends – all congratulating me for what the internet had dubbed my 'Brexit rant'. Many also told me to iron my shirt.

Someone had extracted a 90-second segment from the programme and uploaded it to YouTube, where in the following days it was viewed around four and a half million times. It was flattering and unnerving. I got lucky. My allotted portion of internet fame was not spent in the stocks. The viral dice came up with a double six and I won a few days of approval from strangers, but it could just as easily have been snake eyes, some slip of the tongue, notoriety, and the digital pillory: days of abuse, insistence on apology, retraction, demands for my resignation.

Also, I didn't like the designation of a 'rant'. It is a common vanity among newspaper commentators to picture ourselves as information artisans, whittling opinions with finely pointed words, not fulminating wildly. But the race for a digital audience doesn't favour nuance. Even-handed evaluation plods limply behind monomaniac certainty.

I doubt my performance changed a single mind. My YouTube clip flew around the self-congratulating community of people who liked hearing their beliefs played back to them. Somewhere in an adjacent echo chamber, someone else's rant*

---

* Skilled guests have worked out how to game a TV appearance with the conscious intent of generating a viral message like the one I produced by accident. This practice has also spread to the House of Commons, where MPs will stand, ostensibly to ask a question, and deliver a mini oration for their staff to upload to Facebook. Nigel Farage pioneered this technique as a member of the European Parliament, using the assembly as a stage to deliver anti-Brussels harangues for the gratification of an audience back in the UK that would never ordinarily watch parliamentary proceedings in Westminster, let alone Strasbourg.

was spiralling virally out to millions of people who believed the opposite.

The call from *Question Time* came first thing on the following Monday. My viral glory had reached the attention of producers, always on the lookout for lively panellists. They wanted to know if I could replicate my rant on other issues for the BBC's most-watched current affairs programme. The problem was that I didn't have a fuller menu of hot-and-spicy takes. I felt strongly about Brexit, but even then there was scope for indecision. I couldn't even demand a second referendum without fretting over the offence caused to Leave voters (also I worried the result would be the same as the first one).

I had failed the *Question Time* panel selection process before. Each time it goes the same way. A producer asks for my stance on a range of hot-button topics, and I fail to be succinct.

Welfare, for or against?

It depends. There is a fair critique of cash payments used as a social anaesthetic with no accompanying mechanism for getting their recipients back on their feet. But that argument can be cynically mobilized to justify withdrawal of support from people who face desperate poverty without it. Maybe there is a path of reform that leads to a more financially efficient and socially effective outcome without recourse to dehumanizing rhetoric . . .

Hmm. What about immigration control?

It depends. It isn't politically viable or socially responsible to have unmanaged borders. But stoking anxiety about migration into a national neurosis, often suffused with xenophobic aggression, makes it impossible to have a reasonable discussion about criteria for entry and numbers . . .

On it goes like that, on the one hand, on the other hand, everything depends, until consensus is reached that I should not appear on *Question Time*.

In 1936, *Esquire* magazine published an essay by F. Scott Fitzgerald, whose writing career had by then slid well below its *Great Gatsby* peak. It was titled 'The Crack-Up' and described, among other topics, the author's struggle with depression, mental breakdown and dread of failure. The opening paragraph contains its most famous line: 'The test of a first-rate intelligence is the ability to hold two opposed ideas in the mind at the same time, and still retain the ability to function. One should, for example, be able to see that things are hopeless and yet be determined to make them otherwise.' I like the overall sentiment but disagree with the opening clause. I don't think the ability to function with two opposed ideas in mind is limited to first-rate intelligence. Most people do it at some point, although we might not be conscious of the dissonance.

The most famous technique for managing contradiction into a harmonious political mindset is the one that George Orwell described in *Nineteen Eighty-Four* as doublethink:

> To know and not to know, to be conscious of complete truthfulness while telling carefully constructed lies, to hold simultaneously two opinions which cancelled out, knowing them to be contradictory and believing in both of them, to use logic against logic, to repudiate morality while laying claim to it, to believe that democracy was impossible and that the Party was the guardian of democracy, to forget whatever it was necessary to forget, then to draw it back into memory

again at the moment when it was needed, and then promptly to forget it again.

I first read *Nineteen Eighty-Four* as a teenager (a year or two after the actual 1984) and failed to understand doublethink. I had not then had the infuriating experience of arguing with fanatical ideologues. I had not yet witnessed the feat of mental alchemy by which some people seem able to dissolve the complex, messy base metal of reality into the liquid gold of pure resolution.

In doublethink, the contradiction is conscious, but somehow sublimated to serve a higher, uncomplicated truth. The hot iron of moral righteousness smooths out the logical wrinkles. Orwell describes a triumph of the will to be sure of oneself in pursuit of an agenda. Fitzgerald was getting at something else – paralysis of will in a state of ethical uncertainty.

Democracy has to contain the paradox that people who are contradicting each other can be simultaneously right about something, or right enough. The paradox is resolved by recognition that no one has a monopoly on the knowledge required to achieve the perfect outcome, so the best available one is reached by negotiation. That means considering the validity in a rival perspective long enough to test whether it demands calibrating one's own.

This is not the same as moral relativism, where anything is right if enough people demand it. Nor does it require surrender to the post-truth scrum where facts are determined by control over the media. It is an acknowledgement of imperfection and a willingness to admit that even the most cherished views we have, the sacred beliefs, should be vulnerable to refutation by evidence.*

As a theory, that is all splendid, which is to say it is sullied on contact with the real world. In practice, not all political opinions are equal in a democracy. Some are just lies. Some make violence a justified tool in pursuit of a goal. That is a harder paradox. Democracy tolerates anti-democrats in its midst. It must manage a tension between the duty of respect for diverse opinions and a duty of self-preservation.

(ii) The fallacy of symmetry

Ambivalence is not always a political virtue. (I'm ambivalent about it.) To govern is to choose, as the saying goes. Leaders have to be able to settle on imperfect options and campaign for them with conviction. MPs have to sometimes bury qualms and feign enthusiasm to campaign for policies they don't love if they are persuaded that the alternative is worse. (That psychological manoeuvre gets easier if the alternative means losing their seat or winding up in opposition.)

There is no 'it depends' option on the ballot paper. I don't blame broadcasters for wanting guests with distinct opinions. It wouldn't always be a public service to serve audiences with a tepid mess of nuance porridge. To vote is also to choose and to facilitate the choice; it helps to hear cases for and against articulated crisply.

---

* Even in science and maths, where truths are more fixed than politics, a theory is confirmed not by looking for reasons to believe it but the opposite. Only when avenues of disproof have been exhausted can it be said that the thesis stands.

I have always envied people who can declutter their political calculations, simplifying the equation until it spits out a solution. I tend to keep adding variables. I get bogged down in dilemmas and paralysed by equivocation. Exploring the finer points of a question can be rewarding, but people also want answers. The ability to repress self-doubt in politics is a skill and a trait among great leaders. But it's also common to idiots and megalomaniacs.

Some people are temperamentally more argumentative than others. I am conflict-averse. My idea of an enjoyable political discussion, finding and expanding points in common, would not only make boring viewing; it would fail to satisfy the UK regulator's obligation to show balance.

Ofcom rules mandate that positions from across the political spectrum be afforded air time. The BBC augments that stipulation with an in-house duty to represent racial, gender and regional difference across the UK. The aspiration is not easy to meet simultaneously on every axis of difference. An all-white, all-male panel can cover a wide range of ideological opinions. An ethnically diverse one can be skewed in favour of incumbent government or opposition. And whatever the broadcasters do to adjust the levels of representation, someone will feel excluded. Social media will light up with accusations of bias and conspiracy.

The BBC is an imperfect referee, but it doesn't take much exposure to the partisan frenzy that is US cable news to appreciate the benefits of a system that tries to enforce balance. (The same distinction operates in reverse with newspapers, where the main US titles venerate impartiality, even if they don't always achieve it, while Fleet Street is a carnival route for opinion masquerading as news.) But balance is not a defence against polarization. It is not the same as impartiality, which implies dispassionate retreat from rival arguments to evaluate their merits by some rational criteria. By contrast, balance can be achieved with two equally emotionally overwrought but symmetrically extreme views. The resulting discussion will not illuminate the topic under debate, and it will exclude the large segment of the audience that occupies the under-represented middle ground; the people whose answers begin 'It depends . . .'

The requirement of balance can in that way generate artificial demand for polemical minority opinions. I once took a panicky call from a producer whose guest had dropped out of a debate on badger culling.* They had someone who was pro-badger and needed a balancing view. Could I maybe summon up some synthetic hatred for these nocturnal mammals? (They are vicious creatures, but I couldn't agitate for their slaughter without knowing the arguments for and against, not even for a fee.)

Striving for symmetry in every argument means matching any opinion with its opposite in a way that implies equivalence. That is not a safe premise. It also presumes the two sides are drawing their debating points from a commonly recognized reservoir of basic facts. When the facts themselves are in dispute, or when one side makes up its own facts and refuses to engage on other terms, the requirement for balance becomes a mechanism for legitimizing extremism and misinformation.

For years, the BBC would 'balance' scientists with deniers when the news covered some report on the ravages of global

---

* The government wanted their numbers reduced to limit the spread of bovine tuberculosis, for which apparently they are a conduit.

heating.* During the COVID pandemic, anti-vaccine views were aired on *Question Time*. The defence is that people who hold minority opinions are entitled to have those views represented by the national broadcaster for which they pay. The counter-argument is that a wider public interest is served by denying dangerous attitudes an amplifying platform.

The dilemma is as old as democracy itself. What rights of free speech are protected for the expression of beliefs that can plausibly be said to threaten social harm? And how can that boundary be enforced? Who is to decide when a radical idea is so dangerous to democracy that its exponents need silencing, even if no law has been broken in its articulation?

In analogue times, there was a view that the weakness or menace of extreme politics would be flushed out by appearance on mainstream platforms. That worked in 2009, when Nick Griffin, leader of the far-right British National Party, was invited, amid much controversy, to appear on *Question Time*. He floundered, swerving between creepy sycophancy and playground strop. He later complained that he had been traduced by the London audience – 'a lynch mob' recruited from the liberal burghers of the ethnically diverse capital. The appearance did his cause more harm than good. But social media was in its infancy then. Griffin was not skilled at manipulating mainstream

---

* In April 2018, Ofcom ruled against the BBC over complaints about an interview with Nigel Lawson, the former Conservative Chancellor, whose political dotage consists largely of climate change denial. Lawson had claimed that 'official figures' showed declines in recent temperatures and that the UN Intergovernmental Panel on Climate Change said there had not been an increase in extreme weather events over the past decade. It wasn't true, and the BBC conceded that it should have challenged the claims more robustly. But Lawson is a peer of the realm, a statesman. His grandeur brought an opportunity to invent stuff on air.

opprobrium to his advantage, as more technically adept provocateurs have subsequently been able to do with their own digital channels.

A crowd on social media can change the terms of debate much faster than an analogue audience ever could, and at lower cost. That adjustment in the balance of power is not inherently bad. Journalists should care what audiences think, and the groupthink in established media, staffed with people from similar backgrounds, needs challenging. But it isn't always easy to separate feedback from intimidation. Newspapers and broadcasters that use social media traffic as a barometer of public engagement and the national mood are easily steered into ideological niches by whichever anti-bias vigilantes happen to be making the most noise online.

No news organization will admit to having its agenda dictated by the mob. But that doesn't rule out subtle editorial submission, much of it unconscious, to avoid grief. When you can anticipate with confidence that a certain action will be met with a hurricane of hateful reaction, it is almost impossible not to flinch in advance.

Every moment of hesitation, wondering whether it is really worth the hassle, is a step towards self-censorship. Digital vigilantism works by raising the cost to journalists and institutions of expressing certain views. I have felt this at a personal level. I know, for example, that even just reporting the existence of doubts about the wisdom of Scottish independence brings in a vast haul of irate correspondence from 'cybernats' who consider it impertinent of me, an Englishman, to have brought my ignorant colonial attitudes to a debate reserved exclusively for Scots. Knowing it will happen every time doesn't stop me writing about the subject, but even if you make an active decision to ignore criticism, the effort of steeling yourself for the inevitable barrage and mentally rehearsing responses is a tax on dispassionate judgement.

The ferocity of objections infiltrates the process of formulating a reasonable argument. It doesn't necessarily make you more accommodating. More often it has the opposite effect. Having to brace yourself in advance to repel all the angry things that will be said about you leads to a more assertive, pungent pre-emptive rebuttal. That is also a distortion of the argument, albeit not in the direction your critics want. It is hard to consider the underlying merits of a cause – the case for Scottish independence, for example – while also donning mental armour in anticipation of attack. That is part of the machinery of polarization.

The most unhinged advocates of a cause attract the most attention, generating an intolerant backlash and so entrenching the very biases they claim to be opposing.

(iii) Sense and censoriousness

Balance in politics often refers to an even distribution of weight given to rival arguments. But the state of being unbalanced also implies emotional disequilibrium. Some radical ideas can be reasonably argued, and liberal opinions can be asserted with intolerant vehemence.

In twenty-first-century media, the intensity with which an opinion is held has come to serve as a proxy for its value in a debate. The more ardent the feeling, the more deserving it is of attention. The best expression of that tendency is the frequency with which 'outrage' appears as the subject of a headline.

The following examples are the result of typing 'outrage' into Google right now:

Outrage as children's football pitch defaced by mindless idiots

Plan to fly asylum seekers to Rwanda draws outrage

Outrage as restaurant customer charged £10 to eat their own birthday cake

Outrage as Buddhist monk passes out drunk at Thai temple

Outrage as North Carolina medical school backs woke medical school student who deliberately injured patient

Reading further into these stories, it turns out that 'outrage' is shorthand for irate responses on Twitter. A handful of online fulminators will suffice for the threshold of newsworthy outrage to be met.

As noted in Chapter 6, unthinking emotional urgency is central to the social media business model, and anger is one of the most compulsive experiences available online. We don't intuitively think of rage as addictive because it isn't associated with pleasure. If someone synthesized a new drug that induced impotent fury and despair at the state of the world, people would not be queuing up for a dose. (Alcohol can induce those symptoms, but they are not the advertised effect.) But the addictive cycle does not need an enjoyable experience to get rolling. Surges of anger and frustration involve endorphins and adrenaline – hormones associated with thrills and danger – which get people hooked.

Even if you try to avoid contact with ideas and arguments that you know will make you cross, they can be thrust in your face by friends who hate the same things as you and seek solidarity in common affront. Often disproportionate amounts of mental energy are spent rebutting positions online that few people in real life are advocating. The outrage is directed at spectres and hypotheses of what the enemy camp is imagined to believe – or what one side needs its antagonists to believe in order to sustain its own radical vigour.

The writer Helen Lewis compares it to an ant mill:

> Army ants are blind, and so they follow trails by pheromones. This is a great system right up until the pheromone tracks cross, at which point the ants enter a death spiral, marching round and round until they die of exhaustion.
>
> Twitter is journalism's ant mill . . . For the tweeters, there is an opportunity to signal their own position – this is sexism, which I'm against/this is racism, which I'm against – which is then picked up by columnists, who (I speak from experience) are always desperate for topics, particularly at times when one subject is otherwise dominating the news.

It is usually possible to find someone, somewhere on the internet, to conform to a grotesque caricature of the opinion you want to attack. Then the ant mill starts turning. That doesn't mean the targeted opinion – the racism, the sexism – is a fiction. But it does marginalize nuanced views.

Media overvaluation of outrage and its contagious nature has a distorting effect on most political conversations, but it is especially pernicious in discussions about free speech. There is

– or should be – a distinction between opinions that cause personal offence and political views that would undo democracy if imposed by a government.

Advocacy of violence and hatred can be placed in the latter category. That is why many countries ban neo-Nazis and shut down websites that recruit terrorists. But the category of *dangerous* speech can get bloated by outrage inflation if enough people take offence at an opinion because it is perceived as an assault on their identity.

Here another category distinction matters. There is a difference between conditions where a candid exchange of views is difficult because a public arena (digital or analogue) is flooded with intolerant voices, and a political system where freedom is limited because an anti-democratic authority has formal power of control over what can be said. In each case some people endure the unpleasant experience of having silence imposed on them, but that similarity does not mean the two situations describe identical or even equivalent threats to the principle of free speech.

A person in a democracy who is afraid to voice an opinion for fear of being punished by a freelance battalion of digital thought police is not as free as they would like. But their status is not the same as the condition of an anti-war demonstrator in Putin's Russia or a critic of Communist Party rule in China. In one case, speech is constrained by social taboo – an ancient bullying mechanism now turbo-charged by digital technology. In the other case, speech is rendered *unfree* by the operation of authoritarian state repression.

Modern dictators are well aware of the difference, and game confusion between the two. In March 2022, Putin passed laws banning the distribution of 'deliberately false information' about the army and its actions in Ukraine. The category of 'fake news' included any description of the war as a war. Russian law insisted on 'special military operation' as the official euphemism. Misnaming it carried a potential penalty of 15 years in jail. Journalists have been jailed and newspapers shut down. That is what an unambiguous threat to free speech looks like.

Although the Russian language has a perfectly valid Slavonic word for 'fake', in the sense of counterfeit or artificial, for 'fake news' the Kremlin prefers an anglicized term – фейк (*feik*). This gives the impression that misinformation is a product imported from the West. It was after all Donald Trump who pioneered the practice of accusing professional journalists of peddling 'fake news' when he didn't like the truth they reported.

Putin took Trump's approach to the next level, calling the truth a lie and banning it by law. That is a higher order of assault on fundamental rights than anything described as 'no-platforming' or 'cancelling' in the context of frothy culture-war debates in democratic societies.

But Putin revels in the fiction that liberalism is now the world's sinister repressive ideology. In a televised address in March 2022, the Russian president cast Western sanctions against his country as an attempt to 'cancel a whole thousand-year culture, our people'.

That formula is part cynical trolling and part paranoid obsession with the eastward advance of permissive social values. Putin would never admit the real reason for the sanctions – his military aggressions and atrocities – but the indignant scorn he summons at invasive moral decay is also sincere. His fear that Russia will be made queer by the West is pathological. As so often with dictators, the sinister overlaps with the absurd. 'Not so long ago, the children's writer J. K. Rowling was also cancelled,' Putin said. He explained that the author had been silenced in the West for failing to 'please the fans of so-called gender freedoms'. He compared the promotion of liberal culture to Nazi book-burning.

Rowling rejected Putin's perverse endorsement, but her antagonists on the culture-war front line took it as vindication. To the uninitiated, the controversy that has flooded Harry Potter fandom with political venom looks abstruse. But it is worth taking a detour through this culture-war minefield. It can help clarify a lot of problems with the structure and style of political debate precisely because so much intensity is focused on a relatively narrow strip of ideological terrain.*

Unlike arguments over flags and pulling down statues, the conflict between gender-critical feminists and trans-rights activists does not track conventional left–right or liberal–conservative fault lines. Right-wing Tories and religious reactionaries take a side, but the underlying intellectual fault line is between different ways of interpreting liberalism.

As is the way of civil wars, it is all the more vicious for dividing people who agree on much else. Many of the ethical impulses behind the opposing arguments are the same, but there is so little common ground in terminology that it is hard even to *describe* the dispute without accidentally taking a side.

Rowling's initial offence was committed on Twitter, where she criticized an op-ed that referred to 'people who menstruate'

---

* For the same reason, the summary that follows is certain to dissatisfy a reader who is thoroughly versed in the intricacies of the dispute. For that, I am sorry.

instead of plain 'women'. The alternative formulation is meant to avoid impugning the womanhood of trans women, who were born with (and still have) male internal organs and therefore do not menstruate.

Rowling was the object of a ferocious digital backlash. She elucidated her views in another tweet: 'If sex isn't real, there's no same-sex attraction. If sex isn't real, the lived reality of women globally is erased. I know and love trans people, but erasing the concept of sex removes the ability of many to meaningfully discuss their lives. It isn't hate to speak the truth.'

That didn't placate her critics. Biological sex as a paramount measure of womanhood is precisely the line that advocates of self-identification – the right to be legally recognized by a gender of personal choice, regardless of status at birth – aim to dissolve. In that view, a trans woman is a woman; a trans man is a man.* Any attempt at caveat or hyphenation is effectively a denial of that person's identity. It is a refusal to accept them as they are and therefore a discriminatory and hateful act.

The debate gets so vicious because both sides derive their claim to moral authority from the liberal tradition of protecting vulnerable groups. They are competing for the same patch of high ground, albeit approaching from different angles.

There is also profound philosophical schism lurking beneath the surface. The foundation of the gender-critical feminist

---

* Although in theory the debate is identical both ways, most of the heat is concentrated on the transition from man to woman. I doubt that indicates a greater propensity for tolerance among men, but rather makes the point that men born with male bodies are unlikely to be physically intimidated by trans men, nor see any erosion of political rights implicit in their acceptance as men. An open-door policy on maleness is no challenge to the accrued advantages of patriarchy. That is not the same with womanhood.

position is more material. It is pregnancy, childbirth, menstruation, the historic use of the penis as a weapon of subjugation. It is body issues that define a centuries-long struggle for emancipation and equality. For trans activists the irreducible core of the question comes down to something more abstract – an ideal of the self as defined in the mind and a consequent right to have protection for that self-expression in law.

Both sides can be right. The political task should be calmly refining the arguments until the precise points of disagreement reveal themselves, then considering how to bridge the gaps as they appear in policy. One such area is sport, since being born with male musculature confers an undeniable competitive advantage. Another is physical vulnerability in single-sex spaces, especially prisons and refuges.

Those challenges should not be insoluble, but the quest for solutions relies on both sides accepting some common definition of where the problem lies. That can't happen if even mapping the location of difference is considered an act of prejudice. If it is transphobic to ascribe meaning to the distinction between biological sex and self-identified gender, for example, there cannot be a debate at all, because one of the primary concepts that defines the whole issue has been declared taboo.

Rowling was anathematized by a swathe of the liberal arts world. Actors whose careers were built playing characters she had devised disowned her. She was made *persona non grata* in an influential subculture. But she was not censored in the way that is practised by authoritarian states. Her views and rebuttals were still printed in mass-circulation national newspapers.

The difference matters when digital technology is changing and confusing the nature of free-speech debate. On the left it is sometimes argued that 'cancel culture' doesn't even exist; that it is a bogeyman invented by conservatives to justify their own repressive impulses.

A further objection is that social dynamics ascribed to left ideology and labelled 'cancellation' are no less prevalent on the right. In June 2021, a story appeared in a number of news-papers about the removal of the Queen's portrait from a student common room in Magdalen College, Oxford. The *Daily Express* dedicated the whole of its front page to the affront. 'How Dare They! Oxford Students Cancel Our Queen' ran the headline.

Matthew Katzman, an American PhD student, was identified as the culprit. He was denounced in print and on the floor of the House of Commons, where Jacob Rees-Mogg called him a 'pimply adolescent' (Katzman was 25 years old). As chair of a student committee, he had allowed a motion to remove the print of Elizabeth II that had appeared only a few weeks earlier. (The sovereign's image was displayed elsewhere in the college.) For that sedition, he was made nationally notorious, and sub-jected to a torrent of abuse that caused him to decamp and complete his studies back in the US.

In the Magdalen case, the offence of 'cancel culture' was just a euphemism for *lèse-majesté*. Conservative MPs who make a great fuss about free speech on campus were happy to vote for legislation in 2022 banning public protest on the flimsy grounds that it might cause a 'public nuisance'.

Most were quiet, too, when police arrested demonstrators for grumbling about the monarchy in the period of mandatory mourning for the late Elizabeth II. Episodes of overzealous and partisan policing combine with poorly conceived statutes to blur the boundary between causing offence and menacing public order, although they are very different categories of behaviour.

There is a further ambiguity over what constitutes oppression in a democracy, where coercion is not a power monopolized by the state. It can be wielded in an authoritarian *manner* within social contexts that are constitutionally free.

It was a social movement that punished Rowling for an opinion that many on the left thought should not be heard. She happened to have the resources and the means to resist, projecting her voice over the heads of her critics. Those defences were not available to Kathleen Stock, a philosophy professor at the University of Sussex, who committed the same doctrinal offence as Rowling but without the celebrity resilience.

Stock is the author of a book challenging the primacy of gender identity over biological sex and maintaining that the latter, being a physical reality, cannot be changed by acts of will. Students campaigned for her removal. Posters appeared around campus, lining walls that Stock had to pass on her way into work every morning. In large capital letters: 'It's not a debate. It's not feminism. It's not philosophy. It's just transphobia and it's not on. Fire Kathleen Stock.'

Another read: 'Kathleen Stock makes trans students unsafe. Sussex still pays her.'

Graffiti to the same effect adorned campus walls. There were stickers, petitions and a barrage of abusive messages to Stock's email inbox.

The university was lukewarm in support. Stock's trade union effectively sided with the protesters against their own member by calling for a university-wide investigation into transphobia. One morning she found the atmosphere of intimidation too overwhelming and, hyperventilating with dread, fled the campus and resigned.

That was not state repression, but within the microclimate of a university campus, the government is not the only source of power, or even the one that has the most influence. Informal cultural structures can operate in an authoritarian *mode*. A socially enforced demand for obedience to an intellectual doctrine on pain of ostracism for dissenters is not *exactly* the same as censorship, but it is still aggressively and illiberally censorious.

(iv) The muddy middle

All societies impose limits, formal and informal, on what is said where and by whom. They recognize taboo words and ban some kinds of publication. No one thinks it is censorship that the BBC doesn't allow swearing on daytime television. Free-speech campaigners don't complain if Facebook takes down jihadi recruitment videos.

Most of our cultural and historical reference points for censorship were set at a time when flows of information passed through a small number of narrow pipes. The state could revoke licences to print. Plays to be staged in British theatres were vetted by the Lord Chamberlain until that role was abolished in 1968.

In the digital age, it is rare for anyone in a liberal democracy to find all possible outlets for their opinion shut down. In the Soviet Union, dissidents had to distribute *samizdat* – self-published works in runs of just a few typed copies or hand-written manuscripts. Social media makes self-publishing a universal practice. There are always alternative channels. The withdrawal of one platform doesn't impose a blanket of complete silence.

Does the existence of alternative channels amount to un-limited freedom of expression? No one is 'cancelled' in twenty-first-century Britain as thoroughly as Mikhail Bulgakov was cancelled by the Soviet Writers Union.

'No-platforming' in one venue doesn't preclude appearance on other platforms. Also, pressure by campus activists to have invitations withdrawn from controversial speakers only works if the organizers yield. They might do so out of fear for the safety of a guest or just because it is less hassle than sticking with the original line-up.

The proper word is intimidation, which is hardly better than official censorship, but it is still important to recognize the distinction. It raises questions about the location of political power in a digital age. What was the authority that punished Kathleen Stock for publishing a deviant opinion? *Where* was it? An inchoate social movement that generates and enforces its orthodoxies virally.

Cancellation is a category of social pressure. Whether it is widespread or potent enough to justify moral panic about the well-being of democracy is a different matter. Conservatives ramp up the menace of cancel culture because it resonates with a vaguer social anxiety about smug liberal elites telling ordinary folk what they are allowed to say and think. It is a drill aimed into the seam of cultural grievance that was mined so effectively for votes in the Brexit referendum and the 2019 general election.

There is also envy of the liberal left's intellectual dominance in the realms of art, entertainment and academia – a reserve of soft power that endures through election defeat and exclusion from national government. It is renewed by those setbacks because the losing side in political combat gets compensation as the heroic opposition underdog in culture.

This is a legacy of 1960s counter-culture, when social liberalism established a near monopoly on (self-)righteous indignation in resistance to forces of uptight, emotionally repressive, mindless reaction. Tired of being cast as the bad guys, the right uses the free-speech argument to turn the tables. It is liberals and the left, they say, who are the bullies, and conservatives who are the victims and martyrs. It was much the same argument in the eighties, when the menace was 'loony left' councils thought-policing library bookshelves.

The left has a zealous, intolerant streak that wants to purge culture that doesn't meet its standards of ideological rectitude. The right has a matching strain of hypocrisy, venerating free speech selectively, happy to wield the censor's pen and the policeman's truncheon over anything that has a whiff of sedition.

There must be a lot of people in the middle who would look at the various culture-war front lines and struggle to take a firm view either way. It depends. Apparently contradictory things can be true at the same time. A trans woman can be a woman and also not a woman in *exactly* the same way that someone born into a woman's body has always experienced being a woman. Britain's historical record of aggressive overseas colonization can require atonement without that bloody legacy invalidating every foreign policy decision and international intervention that a modern UK government makes. Sometimes there is no single fixed position that lines up all of the facts and all of the available perspectives into a neat line, with all the virtue on one side.

Insistence that such lines do exist and militant invigilation of the boundaries online forces a lot of people into uneasy silence. Fear of getting on the wrong side of an angry mob is part of that process. Another is aversion to the kind of company you end up keeping when crossing between culture-war trenches.

'In fighting the Communists one is always embarrassed by one's allies,' wrote Arthur Koestler. In the Cold War, opposition to Stalinists put moderate socialists and social democrats on the same side of the argument as conservatives. (During the Second World War, opposition to Hitler had made Churchill a cheer-leader for 'Uncle Joe' and the Red Army.)

Modern dilemmas aren't quite so stark, but the discomfort can be similar. Liberals who sympathize with gender-critical feminist arguments don't want to agree with right-wing Tories. Moderate Tories who think Britain has some painful reckoning to do with its imperial past don't want to say so if it means harmonizing with slogans of the anti-capitalist left. No one wants to have their political identity defined by the worst person whose views overlap somewhere with their own.

But there is a lot more overlap than is visible in a media landscape that militates against ambivalence and nuance. All the noise is coming from the deep-dug fortified trenches, but there are a lot of us huddled quietly, stuck in the churned-up mud in between.

CHAPTER 8

STUPEFACTION

Ideology is not the product of thought; it is the habit or the ritual of showing respect for certain formulas to which, for various reasons having to do with emotional safety, we have very strong ties and of whose meaning and consequences in actuality we have no clear understanding.

Lionel Trilling

(i) Clap if you believe in fairies

A spy once explained to me how war begins with bureaucracy. He is an ex-spy these days, but will stay anonymous for this story. Let's call him Mark. We were discussing the case of Saddam Hussein and the missing weapons of mass destruction (WMD). The Iraqi dictator's arsenal was the pressing official reason for attacking Iraq in 2003. The invasion was straightforward and, in military terms, successful. Saddam was ousted within six weeks. The subsequent occupation was a calamity.

No stores of WMD were found. On the eve of the invasion, one poll showed 54 per cent of people backing the war. Not only did that enthusiasm wane, but people then forgot they had been up for it in the first place. A few years later, only 37 per cent recalled having been pro-war. The weapons issue was lodged in people's minds because Tony Blair had made it the central plank of a legal and political case for action. There was a dossier, presented to Parliament and the public, using intelligence reports to prove that the threat was imminent.

Later, an allegation that the 'dodgy dossier' had been 'sexed up' in Downing Street caused a ferocious row between the government and the BBC. Blair was not toppled by the controversy, but his authority never fully recovered and his party never forgave him. Trust was lost. A perception took hold that government had been warped by the devious arts of spin and that the war had been sold on a false prospectus; that British and Iraqi lives had been squandered.

To this day, Blair insists he did not lie about the WMD; not deliberately. He sincerely expected chemical and biological arsenals to be found in the desert. My man Mark agrees. Mark worked for the non-proliferation department of one of the UK's secret intelligence services. One of his duties was processing reports from defectors fleeing Saddam Hussein's tyranny. It was a vicious dictatorship and escape to Britain was not easy. The Iraqi regime was sealed from Western eyes, so anyone who crossed over bearing insider info was an intelligence asset. The value of that status to those seeking asylum was not lost on potential claimants. Thus, Mark explained, a market was created for intelligence confirming what the UK government wanted to hear about Iraq and its scary laboratories.

The demand side of that market was generated by a political idea – the threat posed by rogue states – and inflated by a civil service bureaucracy (spies are also civil servants). An Iraqi dissident might escape over the border and make his way to

Turkey, where he would be identified and interviewed by some-one working for UK intelligence.

Maybe the fugitive was a scientist. He had been in labora-tories. What kind of laboratories? Where? What was the equipment? If the answers sounded like the sort of thing that could shed light on a covert weapons programme, the report sent back to London – CX, in spy jargon – would be escalated to the highest levels. If it was really good stuff, it might reach the prime minister. It was rewarding for agents to get the CX that everyone wanted. The spy who found it was praised, perhaps promoted, as was the desk officer who passed it on. Mark described how gratifying it was to send in a report and get a personal note of approval back from Downing Street.

Bureaucracy ramped up the price of WMD stories and Iraqi refugees had motives of their own to supply them. They wanted Saddam to be seen as a mortal threat. (And he was, mostly to his own people and their neighbours. The regime had used chem-ical weapons during the Iran–Iraq War, massacring thousands.)

When the time came to draw up a dossier making the case for regime change in Baghdad, there was a trove of supporting CX. The way Mark told it, the war was founded on a mis-perception generated by dozens, if not hundreds of people over many years. No conspiracy, no wilful deception, but a falsehood fashioned from systemic eagerness to give the right answer to a leading question.

There were, of course, plenty of forces driving the Blair government to war in Iraq that were much more powerful than Whitehall habit, not least the prime minister's strategic con-viction that Britain should always move in lock step with the US on matters of defence and security policy. But once the end goal had been decided, the bureaucracy was set on rails to pursue it, with rational challenge and dissent treated as burdensome costs or irrelevance.

That dynamic is repeated in most big organizations. It happens in business as much as politics. In the commercial sphere, the market should punish a terrible idea even if executives have declared it a good one and the board has nodded along. A marketing department might find ways to promote petrol-flavoured crisps or wearable yoghurt, but the customer who doesn't buy them is always right. In a democracy, elections are meant to perform the equivalent function. A government that has convinced itself to do something that won't work should be set right when the electorate passes judgement. Voters, given a free and fair chance to express themselves, can put a limit on ideological excess.

Ideologies in themselves are not always wrong or bad. They are theoretical systems about the workings of the world that can be applied to social and economic problems, generating political solutions. Without ideology, politics can lack organizing principles and moral purpose. Even the most technocratic, managerial politics needs some goal in mind to be managing towards. Technocracy – the idea that government should be run unglamorously, by experts and technical specialists – can also be ideological. Self-styled moderates who congratulate themselves for their judicious attention to evidence can become so insular in like-minded company and arrogant in dismissal of dissent that they start to sound like fanatics. Blair boasted of a pragmatic ethos. He said his lodestar was 'what works', but the conviction that he alone was qualified to apply that metric rendered it meaningless.

The world doesn't often behave the way ideological models predict it should. An ideologue is someone whose theory collides with reality and demands that reality step aside.

One word for that is stupid. It isn't used much in politics because it sounds cheap, more a term of abuse than a category of behaviour. To accuse a rival candidate of stupidity is to assert one's own superior intelligence, which is arrogant and unattractive. It implies that supporters of that candidate are idiots, which is not a way to win their votes.

But politics needs to reckon with stupidity because it is a significant part of human experience and a cause of many political mistakes. One way to diminish the pungency of the word is to acknowledge that everyone, including the cleverest people, does stupid things all the time. Especially in politics.

Ideology creates perverse incentives for people to double down on mistakes and pay tribute to the mistakes of others. It motivates them to rationalize their way into irrational choices. It is a conveyor belt that speeds reasonable minds away from facts and into faith-based judgements. It values obedience to dogma and sycophancy and the high priests who interpret the dogmas over independent conclusion. It numbs the enquiring brain, diverting resources of intelligence that could be spent on good ideas towards the justification of bad ones.

In authoritarian systems, stupefaction runs riot. There is no electoral safety valve, so central authorities never get the wake-up call to alert them to the stupidity of an idea. Most of the worst atrocities of the twentieth century were enabled by the uninterrupted transmission of a dictator's idiotic notions down through a totalitarian apparatus.

When Mao Zedong decided that communist China needed

to boost its steel production as part of the Great Leap Forward, peasants abandoned their fields and threw their iron pots into makeshift furnaces. It was one of many catastrophically stupid policy decisions that caused a famine in which tens of millions died. The steel that was forged came out too low-grade for industrial use.

Something along the lines of what Mark described to me in the build-up to the Iraq War happened in Russia to persuade Vladimir Putin that Ukrainians were craving liberation from their own government and would embrace the invading army as saviours. Russian military intelligence had fed the leader a diet of news he wanted to hear – that President Zelensky's government was a house of cards, ready to collapse at the lightest touch. Many of those involved have since been purged, but there was no pressure on Putin to straighten out his warped perception of reality in public or, as far as we know, in private.

The stupefying power of ideology doesn't require everyone in the system to be passionate about the founding doctrine, or even to have read it. It is sufficient to know how to demonstrate commitment by sucking up to bosses and mouthing the shibboleths that prove conformity with the creed.

When ideological stupefaction takes hold of an institution, original thinking and imagination become a threat to the power hierarchy. Mediocrity and banality must be promoted to keep the ship stable. A stupefied system helps dim-witted people reach positions of influence. It also empowers those who are intelligent and unprincipled – artful at using their brainpower for the strategic gameplay of manoeuvring in an ideological regime.

When events do not behave as the doctrine says they should,

the ideologue confronts a terrible fear of humiliation. The natural responses are denial and deflection. To admit error would vindicate critics, validating what non-believers have been arguing all along. Ideology comes to the rescue, providing an explanation that also justifies punishment of the infidels. Faithlessness itself must be the reason why the policy isn't working.

That cognitive conveyor belt is at work when Remainers get the blame for Brexit not working as advertised. It allowed Corbynites to explain their hero's lack of mass appeal as the result of smears by his sworn enemies and no fault of his own. It is why nationalists accuse unionists of 'talking down Scotland' when they point out practical obstacles to independence. It is why economists and MPs who supported Liz Truss's wild economic strategy in the autumn of 2022 responded to ensuing market turmoil with the claim that global financial institutions were channelling a rotten 'Treasury orthodoxy' that the prime minister's measures were bravely defying.

Confronted with uncomfortable reality, the ideologue presents a rival reality and demands that it be given equal consideration. Refusal to do so is treated as proof of malicious intent.

The phenomenon has been described by Jonn Elledge in the *New Statesman* as the 'Tinkerbell theory', in honour of J. M. Barrie's warning in *Peter Pan* that 'the moment you doubt whether you can fly, you cease for ever to be able to do it.' In pantomime productions of *Peter Pan*, there is a routine where the audience are invited to save an ailing Tinker Bell by applauding. 'Clap if you believe in fairies,' they are told. The Tinkerbell theory of politics holds that unless you believe – and prove it with hearty ovations – the policy won't fly; the fairy will die. As Elledge wrote: 'It's easy to see why the Tinkerbell strategy would be such an attractive line of argument for those who deploy it: it places responsibility for their own fuck-ups squarely on their critics.'

Clever people will believe in fairies and clap harder to sustain that belief if the alternative is admission that everything they thought they knew about politics is wrong.

(ii) Trollology

There is no shortage of ideology online, although it can't be organized on the old analogue model. The grand doctrines that shaped twentieth-century politics were written down. There were sacred texts to interpret and implement. The extreme ideologies that became the blueprint for totalitarian states were dictated to the people – that is literally what dictators do – and enforced by commissars, sometimes at gunpoint. There was a centralized authority to say what was true to the regime's founding vision and what was deviation.

That doesn't work on the internet, and yet something of the uniformity and intensity of the old ideologies is endemic on social media. The organizational structures may be different, but loose networks haven't disposed of intolerant dogmas in the way that email killed the fax machine.

One of the strengths of the internet is supposed to be its resistance to central control. It connects people in non-hierarchical ways, routeing and processing information through millions of channels via millions of minds. For tech optimists, the network harnesses the wisdom of crowds. It is much cleverer than the old-fashioned, top-down bureaucracy. To pessimists, it looks like a vast motor of stupefaction.

The persistence of ideological conformity in an age of explosive technological pluralism feels paradoxical. It is part of what makes politics in the digital arena so disorienting. Here it is hardest to engage without being drawn into the systemic enragement. It helps to disentangle what is politically extreme and what is just socially obnoxious. And for that task it is also important to unpack what is actually new about twenty-first-century radicalism and what is vintage ideology enjoying a retro revival and digital rebrand.

The convention is to use the 'alt-' prefix to distinguish ideological trends of the internet age from the ideas that pre-date them.* Alt-right is a more established term than alt-left, probably because it has achieved more as a force in politics. The alt-left has been influential mostly in protest movements in Western democracies. It has no electoral trophy to match the propulsion of Donald Trump into the White House. (Digital mobilization might not have been the decisive factor there, but it is hard to imagine the noxious seeds of Trumpism flowering quite so prolifically if the terrain of US politics hadn't been irrigated with so much internet poison.)

It is easier to name effects of the alt-right than to define it as a doctrine. Measured by the causes it has advanced, it is racist, misogynist, homophobic and, ultimately, fascist. Its proponents might not have set out to become those things, although that is hardly an exoneration. A bunch of goofy teenagers in a chat room sharing white supremacist memes are building

---

* The analysis that follows is more skewed to the American experience than the rest of this book. That is an unavoidable consequence of the English-speaking internet having its political centre of gravity in America. UK politics imports the vast majority of its digital trends from there.

a neo-Nazi movement whether or not they think they are doing it with some ironic tilt in the font.

The playful, mischievous element is important in the genesis and self-image of internet extremists. It is the 'alternative' styling that makes them *alt*-right, and is the main element of camouflage that enabled them to flourish in plain sight for years, when a more conventional, analogue Nazi party would have become an object of mainstream alarm.

The Trumpian far right is culturally indigenous to the internet, steeped in a particular idiom of pop-cultural subversion and meme literacy that revels in its own frivolity. It affects harmlessness as a style. Sinister concepts were smuggled inside ridiculous terms and childish in-jokes – Pepe the cartoon frog as an emblem of nationalism; 'Electric Boogaloo'* as a code for anti-government insurrection – that disoriented anyone trying to decrypt some underlying programme. It was hard to pin down the danger in a movement that seemed based on triviality. As Helen Lewis has said, the challenge, especially for journalists writing about this phenomenon, was in recognizing that 'people can be simultaneously cringe, ironic, semi-self-aware *and* dangerous.'

The malicious levity that became a tactical weapon for far-right propaganda grew out of the trolling ethos that emerged in nerdy chat rooms and message boards at the start of the twenty-first century, when social media was in its infancy. It

---

*   The derivation of this one is especially arcane. *Breakin' 2: Electric Boogaloo* was the much-derided sequel to *Breakin'* (released in the UK as *Breakdance*), a movie about a dance craze. It became a running internet joke about unlikely or improbable sequels, and from there a tag for the idea of insurrection as the necessary 'sequel' to either the War of Independence or the American Civil War.

was the native language of 4chan and subreddits – the geekiest, cliquiest forums of the early web – that radicalized a generation of angry young white men, often via paranoid misogyny and a possessive playground view of digital culture (video games in particular) as a boys' realm that would be spoiled by the inclusion of yucky girls.

Those sweaty chambers of prolonged adolescence and resentful virginity incubated the incel (involuntarily celibate) movement. It fused a cult of teenage rebellion that had its origins in liberal counter-culture with white supremacism, creating a roiling mass of self-pitying macho rage.

From those basement barracks emerged digital shock troops for the Trump campaign and its subsequent rampage through America's constitutional order. It was a horde of trolls – a word that has come to be applied to a wide range of obnoxious behaviours but has a particular inflection as a category of far-right provocateur.

A troll is now commonly understood to mean any aggressive or abusive person on the internet, but the line between argument and abuse isn't always clear. There is less ambiguity in death threats and racist abuse, but that is trolling at its crudest.

Many hard-core self-identifying trolls are unwell. A 2014 study that applied personality tests to a sample of over 1,200 prolific online commenters found a correlation between those who trolled deliberately and a 'dark tetrad' of characteristics: narcissism, Machiavellianism, sadism and psychopathy. That kind of diagnosis is not surprising, but nor is it very useful. It is misleading to talk about trolls as if they were a countable set of people. There is a disciplined cohort of maniacs who revel in confrontation, and a wider penumbra of unhappy people who are consumed by fury and easily drawn into dysfunctional exchanges online that deactivate their capacity for empathy.

Even when people think they are being civil, they can come across as trolls. A statement of disagreement that would not be judged malicious on its own feels aggressive to the recipient when it comes in a barrage of thousands. The quality of trollishness might not reside in the content of a comment or the intent behind it, but in the amalgamated intensity of a digital storm.

There is a well-documented 'online disinhibition effect' by which people do things on the internet that they wouldn't dream of doing elsewhere. Anonymity is a large part of that process. But there are more subtle elements to digital inhibition – the absence of visual cues that would normally tell someone they have crossed a line, or that the person they are dealing with is emotionally vulnerable.

One of the signs that told me I had to better regulate my Twitter use was a text message that appeared on my phone late one night while I was engaged in some bitter online squabble. It was from a friend and colleague and it said simply: 'Step away from the keyboard.' At that moment, I had become a conduit for the malignant spirit of trollism.

There is an element of performance in digital interactions that has little equivalent in analogue communication. When someone responds to a post on Twitter, their reply is often crafted in terms that are aimed not at the recipient but at third-party onlookers – the loyal followers who will make up the audience for any partisan brawl that ensues. This is the dynamic behind a lot of 'virtue signalling' – making political statements that ostensibly engage with an issue but are in reality declarations of affiliation to a culture warrior tribe.

Making enemies and vilifying strangers is part of the gamification of digital politics noted in Chapter 6. Having fights online is an efficient way to attract attention. A 2021 US study of 2.7 million social media posts from news media accounts and politicians found that those attacking the opposition were twice as likely to be shared. Another study comparing online and offline debate found that the hostile tone was driven by a few individuals hijacking the thread to raise their own status. Any digital discussion, even a WhatsApp group, can become a microclimate of stupefaction.

The first generation of online trolls, who wore the label as a badge of honour, were interested in mischievous disruption of serious conversation. Their animating purpose was 'lulz' (a corruption of 'lols'; laughing out loud) – a riotous, visceral pleasure at someone else's confusion and distress. Lulz are laughs with the spiteful edge of the crowd at the bully's shoulder, spurring him on to be even more vindictive. The political sport of trolls was 'owning the libs' – picking arguments with earnest liberals online, making outrageous comments, needling for reaction and refusing to engage in good faith, purely to infuriate an antagonist.

Alt-right trolling is nihilistic. It is an aggression against the idea that political differences can be resolved by reasoned debate. It targets people who want to persuade, provoking them into impassioned responses. The troll then revels in the imbalance of power, watching someone take seriously an argument that only exists for sabotage.

Vandalistic spite can also serve an ideological agenda. The technique is to push the boundaries of debate beyond some liberal taboo, and then hastily retreat behind an assertion that it is all meant ironically, as an impish game played on the edge of convention. It is the fiction of *only-joking* racism, supposedly less toxic than the real thing. Beneath the thin membrane of playfulness is literal racism; actual fascism.

There is no question that this has been a conscious far-right strategy. In 2017, the *Huffington Post* published a leaked copy of a contributor's 'style guide' for the Daily Stormer, a neo-Nazi website that boasts of its capability to deploy 'troll armies'. One of the recommendations to contributors is not to be too serious:

Generally, when using racial slurs it should come across as half-joking – like a racist joke everyone laughs at because it's true. This follows the generally light tone of the site. It should not come across as genuinely raging vitriol. That is a turnoff to the overwhelming majority of people.

The technique has a much older pedigree. There is a passage in a Jean-Paul Sartre essay from 1944 on anti-Semitism (*Réflexions sur la question juive*):

Never believe that anti-Semites are completely unaware of the absurdity of their replies. They know that their remarks are frivolous, open to challenge. But they are amusing themselves, for it is their adversary who is obliged to use words responsibly, since he believes in words. The anti-Semites have the *right* to play.

They even like to play with discourse for, by giving ridiculous reasons, they discredit the seriousness of their interlocutors. They delight in acting in bad faith, since they seek not to persuade by sound argument but to intimidate and disconcert. If you press them too closely, they will abruptly fall silent, loftily indicating by some phrase that the time for argument is past.

Alt-right trollism has analogue antecedents. What makes it modern is its evolution through awareness of how toxic those precursor doctrines are to the mainstream.

Ordinarily, being taken seriously would be a goal for any fringe movement – a passport to inclusion. But fascism is sufficiently abhorred in Western democracies that the far right has to postpone for as long as possible the moment of recognition. The genius of its digital iteration was the embrace of malevolent frivolity and wilful *unseriousness*. It laundered its menace through absurdity. That technique was made easier by Western liberal complacency about the resilience of democracy. Confidence that totalitarianism had been left for dead in the twentieth century* allowed a zombie resurrection to wander unmolested through twenty-first-century politics.

(iii) Mind your language

There is a scene in Milan Kundera's first novel, *The Joke*, that captures the experience of arguing with militant socialists on the internet, although it was written in 1967. It is the story of a young student who falls foul of Czechoslovakia's communist regime. The action pivots on an impulsive choice by the narrator,

---

* The ways in which utopian thinking about the internet in its early years boosted that complacency will be treated in Chapter 14.

who is bored and frustrated when his girlfriend goes off to a summer camp run by the youth wing of the party. Her letters, extolling the vibrant optimism of her comrades, show more enthusiasm for the teachings of Marx than for the lover she has left behind. In a fit of jealous pique he sends her a postcard: 'Optimism is the opium of the people! A healthy atmosphere stinks of stupidity! Long live Trotsky.'

When he is hauled in front of the district party committee, he tries to explain that it was a joke, a tease, a way to needle his girlfriend, who took herself far too seriously. That makes his situation worse.

'Tell us now, what is it she takes seriously? Things like the Party, optimism, discipline, right? Are those the things that make you laugh?'

He insists that he dashed the postcard off in an instant and hardly even remembers writing it. The party interrogator says that is no defence.

'How you wrote it is immaterial . . . You could only have written what was inside you. That and nothing else.'

The obsession with mental deviation from doctrine – thoughtcrime, as Orwell named it – is a form of stupefaction to which the radical left is particularly vulnerable. (Its intellectual origins might be traced to Christian traditions of sin that lurks in the heart, punishable by God regardless of whether it is manifest as wicked action.) The Marxist left has always been obsessed with bad words as whistle-blowers on a faulty consciousness. In the twentieth century, that logic was applied to the politics of class. Today it is more commonly used to police discourse on race and gender identity.

Some racist epithets, drenched in historical blood, deserve

to be expunged from casual use.* It is right that people make an effort to be sensitive in the way they use language. It isn't all that hard to avoid egregious offence, but nor is it always straightforward.

In March 2019, Amber Rudd, a Conservative cabinet minister, slipped up in a discussion about the abuse that fellow MPs received online. Noting that misogyny and racism were two big founts of digital venom, Rudd said, 'It's worst of all if you're a coloured woman; I know that Diane Abbott gets a huge amount of abuse.'

Abbott was Britain's first black female MP and has been the target of constant, voluminous, vile and violent abuse. She objected to the adjective 'coloured' – an idiom from a bygone era of segregation and normalized casual racism. It was, she tweeted, 'an outdated, offensive and revealing choice of words'. Rudd apologized swiftly, saying she was 'mortified' by her 'clumsy language'.

People who take offence at racially charged comments generally do so with good reason. Those who have been on the receiving end of subtle racist insinuations their whole lives usually know what they are hearing.† Rudd was wrong to say 'coloured' and right to apologize. But that didn't settle the argument online, because the underlying dispute was about intent,

---

* Whether they should be deleted from the vocabulary of white users in all circumstances – never articulated even in quotations or insulated with layers of contextualizing caveat – is a trickier question.

† This is a lesson I wish the left applied as diligently to anti-Semitism as it does, correctly, to other kinds of racism. One of the irritating features of Labour arguments over Jeremy Corbyn is listening to non-Jews explain why Jews are wrong to be upset and that they are wilfully misinterpreting innocent remarks in order to score political points.

and how much can be extrapolated about a person's inner beliefs and political convictions by parsing the exact words they use.

Lots of people who don't keep abreast of such things, especially in older generations, struggled to see the difference between Rudd's offensive formula – 'coloured woman' – and 'woman of colour', which would have been acceptable in left-liberal discourse. The emphasis is altered by turning a past participle into a prepositional construction. The former defines a person more subordinately by their race. But the grammatical shift is slight for the amount of historical and cultural baggage it is expected to carry.

Rudd's supporters accepted her defence of 'clumsy' language. Her fiercer critics pursued Abbott's line that the ill-chosen word had been 'revealing'. Of what? The implication was that a Tory minister, regardless of whether she thought of herself as non-racist and irrespective of the context in which she was literally in the process of condemning racism in a radio broadcast, had flashed a glimpse of the party's racist soul.

No one but Rudd knows what was happening inside her head, but there is a way for left ideology to work around that lack of data. It is the argument that language is an instrument of power and a tool for exerting control. From there it is a short step to the conclusion that the words we use denote our position in a power hierarchy. In that case, ignorance or accident is not a defence against the charge of using terminology that perpetuates injustice.

That quasi-logic is embedded in arguments about 'safe space' for political debate. Recall the accusation that appeared on posters around the University of Sussex accusing Professor Kathleen Stock of making trans students 'unsafe'. There was no danger that she would literally assault anyone. The danger was a conflation of ideological abhorrence and emotional distress. Stock's *ideas* were causing harm because of the way they made some students *feel*.

The elision of real and metaphorical threat is derived from Marxist theory: capitalism is inherently oppressive; words and ideas that reinforce the apparatus of social injustice are acts of complicity in pervasive violence, ergo equal to violence itself.

Stock answered the charge: 'Whether you feel unsafe and whether you are unsafe are two different things. As philosophers we constantly distinguish between appearances and reality, and my book is not actually making [students] physically unsafe.'

Marginalized groups of people have been literally unsafe in many places throughout history, and remain vulnerable to attack to the present day. Trans men and women are targets of physical assault by bigoted thugs. So the concept of an environment where they might feel unthreatened is important. The question is whether that principle of sanctuary is reinforced by expansion to exclude ideas whose mere expression is treated as an aggressive act. It might instead be weakened when stretched too thin.

The hard left has always had a fixation on correct terminology, with no slack given for the unintentional slip or momentary lapse. It is a by-product of moral urgency. If the mission is social justice and the world is divided into people who are for or against it, there can be no ambiguity. Double meanings, ironies, nuances, jokes all become inherently suspect. Playfulness with language is adjacent to carelessness around the purpose to which language should be deployed. If the work is revolution, fun is ideologically suspect.

That is why the word 'woke' as a collective term for radical left ideas in the twenty-first century is associated with joyless piety as much as any fixed doctrine. It is why the alt-right uses mendacious levity as a tool of provocation, and why it works.

Woke is no longer a useful term to describe a set of beliefs, if it ever was. It first emerged as a positive attribute to describe a state of enlightened awareness of racial injustice. It was then appropriated by the right to decry left-wing revision of history, toppling of statues and general expunging of cultural symbols from national life. Once established as a pejorative term, it was renounced by the people it was meant to describe.

A 2021 opinion poll found that around half of UK respondents knew little or nothing about what 'being woke' meant. Of the other half, opinion was equally divided on whether it was a compliment. Arguments about empire and gender pronouns are way down the list of topics that worry an electorate that is more concerned with heating homes, paying bills and the state of hospitals.*

Any government presiding over economic misery would rather talk about something else, so there was an incentive for Conservative MPs in the early 2020s to reroute conversation towards the apparent scourge of knee-taking lefty agitators disparaging flags and scrawling trigger warnings over the school curriculum.

---

* During the 2022 Conservative leadership election, when culture-war issues were a prominent feature of the debate, one poll of Tory party members – notionally the target audience that was being mobilized around these questions – found that only 3 per cent felt passionately about trans identification issues. Free-speech arguments, framed around 'the right to say what you want, even if it upsets or offends others', were important to 13 per cent.

In the 2022 Conservative leadership contest, Rishi Sunak, steward of Tory economic policy under Boris Johnson, tried to ingratiate himself with his party's grassroots with a promise to 'take on this lefty woke culture that seems to want to cancel our history, our values and our women.'

Most anti-woke politics is a mix of cynical diversion and reds-under-the-bed paranoia. That doesn't mean the ideological phenomenon being caricatured is fictitious. There is a strain of dogmatic politics that is influential in policing terms of debate in liberal and left-wing circles online. It is less potent than its detractors claim and real enough to intimidate anyone who gets into its bad books.

It is hard to pin down because, like the alt-right, it is indigenous to the internet. There is no party authority issuing edicts on whether or not a particular writer or professor has fallen foul of orthodoxy. There is no building where someone wanting to obey the correct thought processes or keep up with the proper terminology can go for updates. The right way to be left emerges organically and is enforced informally.

The alt-left draws its energy from a young, university-educated middle class. That might explain why it prefers battles over gender, identity and race as opposed to the twentieth-century struggle for proletarian emancipation. The organizing hub of struggle has shifted from factories to campus humanities departments.* That isn't to say the alt-left is reconciled to

---

* An alternative term to 'woke' that has utility as a historical place marker is 'the successor ideology'. The phrase was coined by the US writer Wesley Yang to characterize a chapter in the evolution of left-wing thought that emerged from the traditional political liberalism of the post-Cold War era and is in large part a reaction against, it but that doesn't posit much by way of an alternative programme.

capitalism. But it has absorbed more features of the individualist, consumer-oriented societies in which it grew up than it likes to admit. There is a lot more emphasis on personal emotional self-actualization and a lot less clarity about how society will be organized after the revolution than there was when Lenin and Trotsky were the guides.

(iv) A toxic mist

Digital revolution was meant to be the end of clunky, monolithic politics where correct belief is transmitted down the bureaucratic line by diktat. That model has withered, but ideological conformity adapted and survived.

The internet has simply changed the character of old ideologies. Alt-left and alt-right are hybrids. They are the product of cross-pollination as ideas indigenous to the nineteenth and twentieth centuries – nationalism, Marxism – are filtered through a network built to specifications from twenty-first-century globalized capitalism. They are decentralized, unruly, individualist; also intolerant, repressive, stupefying. They are liberal in form, authoritarian in content.

In some respects they go further than authoritarianism, which is a model that can work with relatively passive populations putting up with a single domineering leader. The alt-ideologies rely more on active displays of loyalty. The requirement of believers is a *performance* of belief. The word for that is totalitarian. But it is a paradoxical hobbyist kind of totalitarianism that is casually regimented, part-time yet full-on.

In noting some left–right symmetries, I don't mean to imply moral parity. In recent years, the far right has propelled its candidates into high office in a number of European countries. It has captured the US Republican Party. Russia is an ultra-nationalist troll state with nuclear weapons. The far left today has a lot of ground to cover before it looks like an equivalent threat to anyone apart from people on the right. Conservatives denounce it either because they are in denial about the menace closer to home or because they *are* the menace.

The new online ideologies are also social identities. They are informal tribes held together by attitudes, not parties governed by rules. That is a shift in the way hard-line politics – once a relatively niche pursuit – is felt by the casually engaged citizen. It adds to the alienation of people who might want to dabble in politics without being consumed by it. The barrier for participation is raised because the terms of engagement are so fierce, while the available space for a less frenzied kind of involvement has shrunk.

A lot of argument online feels disconnected from the real world. It has its own virtual dynamics; its own dialect of memes and ephemeral references. But the radicalizing dynamics feed back into analogue politics. The applause of all the Tinker Bell revivalists online reverberates around the chamber of the House of Commons.

Although there may not be an increase in the number of people professing allegiance to a named ideology, politics in the digital age feels more ideologized in a nebulous way. The pernicious mental habits that accelerate people away from reasonable engagement are more diffuse but no less potent. Doctrinaire intolerance is not concentrated on the fringe, or in any one organization, but is dispersed like a fine mist, leaving its stupefying residue on every exposed surface.

CHAPTER 9

JOIN THE DOTS

The man who believes a thing is true because he feels it in his bones is not really very far removed from the man who believes it on the authority of a policeman's truncheon.

E. M. Forster

(i) Order from chaos

When I first lived in Moscow, in the mid nineties, I rented a room from Lidia Sergeevna, a widow in her fifties whose husband had been a mid-ranking Communist Party apparatchik. That status came with an apartment in a much-desired block, set aside for the *nomenklatura* – the Soviet elite – within walking distance of the Kremlin. In one of our first conversations, Lidia told me that her husband had been ugly but kind, and that I shouldn't believe the spiteful neighbours who said she only married him for the apartment.

Lidia and I got on famously, most of the time. We had an understanding reached over shots of cheap Armenian cognac. Getting drunk improved my Russian and allowed her to avoid drinking alone. The only rule was that we didn't talk about religion. She had raised it once and been unimpressed to learn that I didn't believe in God – an offence compounded by my failure, in her eyes, to be authentically English. This had been established, as it so often was in Russia, within moments of being introduced.

'Where are you from?' Lidia asked.

England, I said.

'But clearly you're not English. Look at you, dark and curly-haired. What are you really? Where is your family from?'

I gave the short version. South Africa, but not South African. Lithuania, but not Lithuanian. Jewish . . .

'Aha! So why did you say you were English?'

She wasn't hostile, just glad to have solved the mystery. Maybe a little disappointed, as if she had asked for a Coke and the waiter had brought Pepsi. She was fine with a Jewish lodger, but she had ordered an English one.

One afternoon on my way home, I passed a rally of Russian National Unity, a fringe neo-Nazi party that was active in the nineties. Its headline policy was the expulsion of undesirable ethnicities from the motherland. It wasn't a big crowd, maybe 50 or 60 people; an inner circle of shaven-headed youths, an outer tier of morose pensioners. I hung around for a bit out of curiosity, trying to radiate proud Slavic vibes for my own protection. I picked up a copy of the party newspaper before leaving.

The entire edition was dedicated to exposing 'the Yids' (Жиды in Russian) who were plotting to defile Russia and plunder her natural resources. This was an easy enough con-spiracy theory to promote, because a number of the most prominent emerging oligarchs at the time were Jewish. But the newspaper editorial didn't limit itself to the obvious anti-Semitic angle. It implicated Boris Yeltsin himself, whose real name, according to the author, was Baruch Yeltzer. The president had Russified it to cover Semitic roots. The same article explained how the Soviet Union had been undone by another Jewish infiltrator. His alias was Mikhail Sergeyevich Gorbachev, but by birth he was alleged to be one Moishe Solomonovitch. The whole thing was so obviously deranged, I found it more comic than sinister.

I read the newspaper at the kitchen table, then chucked it in the bin. The next day, I came home to find that Lidia Sergeevna had retrieved it and was poring over the text.

'That stuff is crazy, isn't it?' I said.

'Crazy, yes.' She sounded unsure. 'Maybe. But there is also a lot that makes sense.'

'But you don't want to get rid of all the Jews, do you?'

'Jews are no good,' Lidia said firmly, before adding an emollient afterthought. 'Don't take offence. I don't mean you, of course.'

A pause.

'You're one of the good ones.'

I chose not to let Lidia Sergeevna's sympathy with a mad anti-Semitic conspiracy theory spoil our relationship. She wasn't unusual among Russians for thinking that Jews were all in league with each other. Often it was presented to me as a compliment, as if I should be proud to belong to the slyest, most cunning race, which had outwitted so many nations throughout history.

Anti-Semitism had deep roots in Russia, and the chaos of the nineties created perfect conditions for conspiratorial thinking in a disoriented, demoralized population. The Soviet collapse, a motherland in a state of nervous breakdown, caused fits of Potemkin syndrome.

The world as people had known it was turned upside down, and no one seemed to be in control. None of it made sense in relation to the politics that had come before or the world as it had been taught in schools. People needed an explanation that would put the messy pieces into some kind of order. To someone like Lidia Sergeevna, trying to come to terms with her personal downgrade in the post-Soviet social hierarchy, alongside economic insecurity and wounded national pride, a Jewish plot made as much sense as any other explanation.

It is one of the oldest and most resilient conspiracy theories, with a credible claim to be the progenitor of the whole genre.* The modern form of it was codified in a tract that started circulating in Russia in the first years of the twentieth century as *The Protocols of the Elders of Zion*. That text, purporting to be secret minutes from the first Zionist Congress in Basel in 1897, is still spawning breathless blogs and fanatical Facebook pages 120 years later. In it, the 'elders' reveal their playbook for world domination: enslaving Gentiles with debt, polluting their minds by dictating what appears in their newspapers, manipulating their states through puppet ministers to foment wars, from which the Jews will profit and further entrench their power.

In reality, the *Protocols* was an act of crummy plagiarism, lifted from an obscure French text imagining a dialogue between Montesquieu and Machiavelli. It had been translated

---

* In their book *Conspiracy: A History of B*llocks Theories and How Not to Fall For Them*, Jonn Elledge and Tom Phillips follow the thread all the way back to medieval anti-Semitic blood libels – the idea that Jews ritually murdered Christian children.

and dispersed by Russian reactionary nationalists to help deflect blame for social disorder and political dysfunction away from the tsarist authorities.

It worked. The *Protocols* inflamed the anti-Semitism that was already raging in Russia at the turn of the twentieth century. The libel then spread to Europe and the US. In Britain, it was published as *The Jewish Peril*. *The Times* called it 'a singular little book . . . likely to perturb the thinking public'. In 1920, a version of the conspiracy theory was printed in a newspaper owned by Henry Ford, the automotive industrial pioneer, under the title *The International Jew: The World's Foremost Problem*. Long after its exposure as fiction, the *Protocols* continued to capture political imaginations.

Anti-Semitism excited nationalists and socialists; reactionaries and radicals. The right blamed Jews for fomenting Bolshevism; the left despised them as the puppet-masters of capitalism. In *Mein Kampf*, Hitler praises the *Protocols* as an aid to enlightenment of the masses. Russian fear of Jewish plotting survived the transition from tsarist autocracy to proletarian dictatorship, resurfacing in Stalin's campaign against 'rootless cosmopolitans'.

The same paranoid energy that powered suspicion of a Jewish world government drives twenty-first-century Islamophobia. Much of the underlying demonology is the same – an alien people with an immiscible culture that refuses to dissolve itself into the majority. The alleged method is not political and media infiltration but migration and childbirth, a demographic subterfuge called 'the Great Replacement'. This theory, popular in radical right-wing circles on both sides of the Atlantic and increasingly influential in mainstream conservatism, posits a plot to exploit declining fertility among white people, flooding their ancestral lands with migrants and outbreeding them. All peoples of colour are despised in this doctrine, but Muslims are feared the most.*

Another common target for nationalist conspiracy hunters, especially in Eastern Europe, is the movement for gay and transgender rights, conceived as a plot against national virility. Vladimir Putin is a strong exponent of this particular theory, supported by the teachings of the Russian Orthodox Church.† In the early days of Russia's war against Ukraine, Moscow's Patriarch Kirill gave a sermon in which he explained that gender fluidity was imposed on countries seeking acceptance by the decadent liberal world order. 'Pride parades are designed to demonstrate that sin is one variation of human behaviour,' the head of the Russian Church declared. 'That's why in order to join the club of those countries, you have to have a gay pride parade.'

The conspiracy theory gets a purchase on the popular imagination at times of chaos, which makes it a powerful device for authoritarian regimes wanting to exert control by promising to restore order. The fear springs up organically but is also factory-farmed. The poisonous dynamics of radical ideology described in earlier chapters reach their apogee in conspiracism. Nationalists whose plans have failed need scapegoats. Populist campaigns need unifying theories of decline that will scythe through the unsatisfying calibrations of boring expertise.

---

* Drill deep enough into that well of racist paranoia and pretty soon you encounter neo-Nazis who assert that the true masterminds of the replacement, the evil race in whose hands the migrant hordes are but pawns, are the Jews.

† Also historically an echo chamber for Russian nationalist anti-Semitism.

Imagined conspiracies have a thrilling potency because they imitate the cognitive satisfaction of independent discovery. They induce an insidious kind of stupefaction that feels like cleverness. The process of joining the dots, finding the patterns in events, animates the psychological need to feel in control, to weave order from disorder and make sense of the world inside the mind.

Not every theory is all-encompassing. Some are less ambitious. They fuss in narrow cul-de-sacs of history. And not everyone who subscribes to one cockamamie story buys the whole set. Someone might think the Apollo moon landings were faked but still take their COVID vaccine; or suspect MI6 of assassinating Princess Diana while stopping short of thinking it was done on the orders of a Masonic world government. But if you take an interest in any of the minor paranoias and follow the leads down the internet rabbit holes, letting the YouTube algorithm nudge you along the sweaty channels, you quickly arrive at one of the meta-conspiracies. Health scares about mobile phone masts are rarely more than a few clicks away from the Illuminati, the Committee of 300, the lizard people, the Rothschilds, the Elders of Zion.

(ii) There has to be reason

In late January 2022, Boris Johnson was in trouble. Stories had begun to emerge of parties in Downing Street when the country had been locked down to prevent the spread of COVID. Public fury was making Tory MPs anxious about their future election prospects. The prime minister's denials sounded, as usual, more like obfuscations and deflections.

In one particularly testy exchange in Parliament, Johnson tried to discredit Keir Starmer by bringing up his previous career as Director of Public Prosecutions. In that role, Johnson alleged, Starmer had spent his time 'failing to prosecute Jimmy Savile'.

It was a bizarre non-sequitur, and untrue. Savile was a prolific paedophile whose marauding offences across decades had been ignored and covered up by institutions – the BBC, most culpably – that had benefited from his celebrity power and status as an icon of charitable benevolence. But the failure to bring him to justice before his death in 2011 could not be connected to Starmer. Or not reasonably. There was a way to do it with the circumstantial insinuations and rhyming pseudo-logic that piece together conspiracies. As a former director of public prosecutions, the Labour leader had once occupied a position of influence in the criminal justice system that had failed to catch and punish a villain. Two dots easily joined.

With his back against the wall, Johnson lashed out, flinging the foulest mud that came to hand, dredged from the most noxious political sewer. It was the same one that Donald Trump played in, where right-wing populism sloshes around with tales of QAnon – the vast, rococo edifice of sinister association that traces COVID vaccines, immigration, gun control, banks and liberal politicians back to a cannibalistic, Satan-worshipping, child-abusing secret world government.

Days later, as Starmer was leaving Parliament, he was accosted by a mob, shouting 'traitor' and 'paedophile protector'. Johnson's dirty deflection had done its job.

I first came across this genre of conspiracy theory in February 2014. I remember the date because I was covering a by-election in Wythenshawe and Sale East, a suburb of Greater Manchester. I was canvassing opinion in a café, where a middle-aged woman told me that her family had always been Labour voters, but she was switching to UKIP. She had many reasons, but the most urgent, she said, was explained on a website that I should check out if I was interested in what was *really* happening in politics.

I checked it out. The site was crudely designed and unpersuasive, except to someone with a will to be persuaded. MPs were named alongside news reports about paedophile rings and failed prosecutions, coupled with dates and cryptic quotations. If the dots were arranged in a certain pattern, omitting all extraneous context and circumstance, a picture of sinister complicity emerged. Secret connections and hidden power networks.

I saw the theory spread and mutate over the subsequent months and years, gaining currency with a wider audience, cross-fertilizing with different species of conspiracy. In November 2014, the Metropolitan Police launched Operation Midland to investigate claims by a man called Carl Beech (posting online under the pseudonym 'Nick') that a number of high-profile and well-connected Establishment figures – politicians, peers, military officers – had committed a range of horrendous crimes, from child abuse to murder.

The cause was taken up by MPs and campaigning investigative journalists. The homes of alleged perpetrators were searched, computers taken, lives turned upside down, reputations destroyed and no evidence unearthed.

Operation Midland concluded in March 2016. The allegations had all been false. Beech himself was found to be a liar and a child sex offender. In 2019, he was sentenced to 19 years in prison. Meanwhile, the idea of a 'VIP child abuse scandal' continued to flourish online. Naturally, for adherents of the theory, the decision not to prosecute confirmed that the Establishment was covering up the truth. How could the police be trusted to investigate when they were in on it too?

That is the unbreakable seal on any conspiracy theory, the link at one end of the chain that joins to the first segment to form a perfect circle of pseudo-logic: if everyone in power is part of a plot to conceal the truth, anyone who is close to power will have reason to fear the truth being told and so will deny it. The absence of proof becomes more evidence confirming the theory.

A powerful impetus to the paedophile conspiracy theory in Britain was that there had been a far-reaching cover-up involving a famous perpetrator whose fingerprints were all over national institutions. It was a real scandal that exposed genuine deficiencies in the system. There was not far for the spark to jump from justified dismay and fury to illumination of something even more sinister, organized and purposeful.

Purpose is the key ingredient that elevates dysfunctional government and bad luck into supreme malevolence with a master plan. Appalling things on a sufficient scale demand explanations. It is not satisfying to be told that they *just happen*, or that no one can be sure why. Someone has gained from it, so someone must have devised it for gain.

The psychological appetite for motive and meaning made the pandemic an especially fertile time for conspiracism. It had all the ingredients. An invisible threat appeared suddenly and with obscure origins in China, an authoritarian state where official information was unreliable. The public health measures required to combat the spread of the disease were draconian, and looked just like the repressive measures that a tyrannical regime would introduce to suffocate freedom.

Citizens were confined to their homes, where they became increasingly reliant on the internet for information and increasingly cut off from diverse social and cultural contacts. To cap it all, the government kept changing its message, U-turning on its policies and cheating in its procurement procedures, compounding the impression that nothing was fixed and the appearance of events was a facade. Anxiety, confinement, mystery and political opacity – a hothouse for breeding paranoia.

It would be wrong to cast everyone who was reluctant to receive a COVID-19 vaccination as part of the conspiracy theory movement. There was a spectrum. It started with a sensible portion of wariness about the competence of government. It is not unreasonable to query the ethics of multinational pharmaceutical companies.*

A good way to nudge someone towards the wackier end of that spectrum is to presume they are already there and accuse them of irrationality, when in their own mind they are committed to rational scepticism. That is a lesson anyone who debates a vaccine resister learns quickly. The argument goes round in circles and usually ends up amplifying frustration and

---

* In 1996, Pfizer ran what amounted to experimental trials of an anti-meningitis drug in Nigeria, administering it to children. Previously, Trovan, the new antibiotic, had only been tested on adults, with evidence of serious side-effects. Within a month, 11 children given the drug had died; others had severe, disabling reactions. Parents said they had not been informed enough to give meaningful consent. It is hardly surprising if that legacy left some people disinclined to consider Pfizer a trustworthy distributor of mass injections.

suspicion on both sides. The obstacle is usually misunderstanding about what, in essence, is really being disputed.

In the case of COVID, most arguments weren't ultimately about the efficacy or safety of the drugs. That was where the conversation started, and the common vocabulary gave an illusion of shared terms of reference. But science, and what it counsels, is really a proxy for something more fundamental to the cohesion of a democratic society. It is about trust and what constitutes a valid authority.

Both sides will bring something they call 'evidence' to the debate. The real dispute is over the reliability, sources and methodologies behind that evidence. Someone who is prepared to believe that their government *might* be sneaking poison into their children's veins is unlikely to be swayed by counter-arguments drawn from official government statistics.

That road might lead to irrational places, but it gets there in increments that resemble the mechanics of rationality. Conspiracy theory is different to religion in that way. The beliefs may be held with similar fervour, and the style of proselytizing often resembles God-fearing zeal. But the mental apparatus that must be climbed to attain great heights of conspiratorial delusion is *rationalistic*, even when the conclusions eventually reached are wild.

If the anti-vax movement was hostile to the scientific method in principle, it would not have put so much effort into imitating the idiom of peer review and laboratory research. The YouTube videos and memes that spread misinformation co-opt the style of bona fide sources, cherry-picking bad conclusions from good data to poach the credibility of accredited expertise. They lean hard on the testimony of the few nurses and doctors who get on board with the dodgy science. They love a lab coat. Even the people in the deepest rabbit holes, who think the injections send government microchips to the brain and rewrite DNA, often try to make their point with numbers and charts.

The element that distinguishes real science from pseudo-rational imitation is the embrace of uncertainty. It is a feature of any genuine enquiry for facts, but abhorrent to the conspiratorial mind. A proper pursuit of truth will admit the difficulty of knowing anything with 100 per cent conviction. The honest scientist recognizes a margin of error – a gap into which the conspiracy theorist will crawl. With any medicine, the risk of harm is rarely nil. Some people will have adverse reactions; some of those reactions will be strong. The risk of a severe allergic response to the Pfizer jab is around one in 90,000, or 0.001 per cent. A very small number, but not zero. And to the committed conspiracy theorist, a whole heap of fear can be extracted from a tiny nugget of doubt.

That is the difference between actual scepticism and the affectation that calls itself sceptical but is really a determination to believe something in spite of evidence to the contrary. The Eurosceptic is not really sceptical about the EU; the climate sceptic is not sceptical about climate science. They are hostile and looking for reasons to reinforce that hostility. They are using rationality to buttress the sacred beliefs that are embedded in their political identity.

The variable is whether the founding premise of an argument is open to challenge. What is someone setting out to prove, and how prepared would they be to accept a disappointing conclusion if that is where their inquiry leads? The person who sifts the news for signs that the government is up to something sneaky will always be able to assemble the case. The argument feels all the more compelling when we have made the connections ourselves, solving the riddle. There is that gratifying mental click of a jigsaw piece finding its right place, except the picture is a fantasy.

There is pleasure in finding logical connections, but that is exactly the problem. A conclusion driven by what *feels* right will prioritize cognitive comfort. Actual logic doesn't always reassure. It hurts when a logical conclusion intrudes on a comfortable prejudice.

Joining dots is an unreliable method for analysing things that might be related in non-linear ways. Before the development of modern astronomy, people saw patterns in the stars, drew pictures and told stories about what the constellations meant. The human mind likes stories that project meaning onto a world that can seem terrifying without one, which is why astrology is still popular. Intimidated by the disorderliness of the universe and our helplessness in the face of unfathomable forces, it can be reassuring to read that money worries will ease once the moon enters Sagittarius.

Politics has always exploited that frailty. In any campaign, stories beat graphs; confidence trumps doubt; definite is better than probable; simple answers cut through nuanced inference; primary colours beat shades of grey.

There are evolutionary reasons why we are so easily seduced by storytelling. The survival of our primitive ancestors depended on the ability to learn quickly from anecdote and vivid representation – wisdom was received by word of mouth and made memorable with gestures or music. Only later did we develop the capacity to collect information, and then start processing data from which measured analysis might follow.

The brain's hunt for causal connections and dot-joining to banish mystery is the origin of superstition. If it rained after the tribe did a dance, it was worth dancing again when rain was needed. Superstitions heaped upon each other were then elaborated into religions. There is some disagreement among evolutionary scientists as to why that habit has proved so tenacious, but few dispute that a religious frame of mind conferred survival advantages down the line, and that kept the habit of magical thinking in the gene pool. A tribe that develops ritual hand-washing might be less prone to disease than one that eats where it shits. The society whose priests make paradise sound like the first prize in a race to martyrdom will have more motivated warriors than one whose soldiers are afraid to die.

(iii) Pulling the strings

The storytelling imagination is always active, shaping politics and boosting some candidates ahead of others. But there are economic and social circumstances in which joining narrative dots becomes a more prevalent mode of analysis.

One reason that conspiratorial thinking has such traction in Eastern European politics can be traced back to the experience of one-party communist rule. Marxism–Leninism sold itself as a scientific account of human behaviour. It was an engineering manual for the development of a better society. That approach defined political and historical analysis from the classroom to the politburo.

The Communist Party view depicted the world unfolding as

a technical process, driven by historical laws of class conflict that could be studied in the same way as gravity or fluid mechanics. In that conception, nothing happens by accident. Politics is the expression of rationally deducible forces. If the system doesn't behave in line with the forecast, the only logically admissible reason is systemic opposition. The sabotage must be organized and engineered on a scale equivalent to the grandiose ambitions of the theory that is failing.

That is the tradition in which Putin had his political apprenticeship as a KGB operative. If liberal societies are an unruly mess of forces with no central control, how could they be getting the better of Russia? The only explanation is that the mess conceals some strategic coordination.

The need for stories that dispel confusion grows in proportion to the gap between ideology and reality. Conspiracism makes a splendid bridge between the official account of what was supposed to happen and how things turned out. That was true in the Soviet era and in the post-communist places where market reforms went wrong. It was true in the West when the promise of steadily rising prosperity and opportunity turned to stagnation and insecurity. It is true when a government promises that the nation will 'take back control' of its destiny, only to deliver years of feeling buffeted and assailed by events at home and abroad.

In *Voodoo Histories*, a thorough debunking of many conspiracy theories, David Aaronovitch makes an important observation about the economic and political climate in which *The Protocols of the Elders of Zion* first went viral to an international readership. It was, he notes, the aftermath of the First World War – a cataclysm that was all the more traumatic because it brought an abrupt end to the preceding era of relative peace and prosperity driven by trade liberalization and migration. Economic historians describe that period from around the 1870s to August 1914 as the first globalization.

There is an obvious parallel with the present era: the shock of good times ending; the bursting of a complacent bubble; the nationalistic backlash against liberal globalism. Under the circumstances, it would be surprising if conspiracy theories were *not* flourishing on the radical underbelly (and spreading across to the mainstream overbelly) of British politics in the twenty-first century.

Part of the appeal is the idea that someone, somewhere is in charge. It isn't a pleasurable reassurance, more an assertion of control, like probing a toothache with your tongue to find the exact point that triggers a spasm of pain.

Although the conspiracy story itself is dark and pessi-mistic – bad people plotting wicked deeds – buried in the misanthropic sludge is a kernel of optimism about the capacity of politics to achieve things. The embittered paranoiac cannot destroy the component of their cynicism that was once ideal-ism. That is why they are often so evangelical about their theories. If someone really believes that the Establishment controls everything, why even bother complaining about it. Why did anti-vax demonstrators line the streets holding placards warning of the perils of government injection and pleading with passing motorists to open their eyes to the '*plan*demic'? The will to proselytize is a form of compassion to save lost souls.

As Aaronovitch writes: 'The paradox is that, seen this way, conspiracy theories are actually reassuring. They suggest that there is an explanation, that human agencies are powerful and that there is order rather than chaos. This makes redemption possible.'

Another, more mundane driver of conspiracism is that in politics, conspiracies do happen. The very nature of the business involves some secrecy, plots and attempted cover-ups. Governments would naturally prefer to keep the full extent of their incompetence or corruption hidden from voters, but it can't usually be done for long, and the more complex the plot, the likelier it is to unravel. Watergate is the best-known example of a big scandal in the genre close to bona fide conspiracy, and even then the plot stumbled along as a concatenation of accident and stupidity.

Also, there was a whistle-blower, villains went to jail and the president resigned. That's a pretty crap conspiracy.

In totalitarian states, it is relatively easy for governments to deceive enough of their populations to keep bad deeds out of view. But if democratic governments were capable of secret machination on anything like the scale alleged in the crackpot corners of the internet, they would not be so routinely ridiculed for elementary incompetence. If the pandemic really was planned, the government presumably also prepared its own displays of hapless unreadiness, perhaps as a decoy. Maybe Johnson's flagrant inability to make timely decisions was an ingenious act designed to maximize the death toll and make it look like a political accident.

Jonn Elledge and Tom Phillips put the point neatly: 'We have plenty of evidence for how competent governments, corporations and powerful people in general actually are. The answer is "not very". Which rather raises the question of why they suddenly become almost infallible as soon as they're doing conspiracies.'

It doesn't take many encounters with senior politicians to realize that few of them have the organizational skills or discipline required to fake a 9/11 or bluff a moon landing. Even if ministers wanted to insert secret microchips into everyone by means of a bogus vaccination programme, they would probably screw up the tender and order syringes with the wrong gauge. Downing Street aides describe a constant, frantic and losing battle to keep one step ahead of the following morning's headlines. As one veteran of No. 10 once told me: 'If people knew how disorganized it all was, they would be even more worried.' The truth – that no one is really in charge – can be harder to take on board than the idea that someone is pulling the strings.

(iv) Hiding in plain sight

For journalists working in Westminster, including me, a reliable rule of thumb when things go wrong is to presume cock-up as a likelier cause than conspiracy. Applying that rule puts us on the wrong side of the line for anyone hoping to draw malfeasance out of mishap.

But the amateur sleuths of sinister plots have a contradictory relationship with 'mainstream media'. Our output is a necessary supply of clues about the conspiracy, but we are not trusted as sources in any other respect. A common complaint on social media, in emails and letters to journalists is that we are failing to report significant things. The evidence of those things is submitted for our attention in the form of reports we have written about them.

It is relatively easy to refute the claim that something has been kept secret when it has been broadcast by the BBC. The harder charge to rebut is the broader allegation of cultural affinity, shading into complicity, between media people and politicians. The cosiness can be real enough (more on this in Chapter 11). Also potent is the observable chumminess between business and government that short-circuits mechanisms of democratic accountability (coming up in Chapter 12). A pattern of mutual back-scratching between wealthy elites and ministers can't be written off as the product of overactive imagination. The 'VIP lane' to expedite procurement of equipment to fight the pandemic was policy, not paranoia.

David Runciman makes this point in *How Democracy Ends*: 'Representative democracy does empower elites and they do conduct much of their business behind closed doors. Any political system that trumpets the value of openness while holding on to its secrets will create the space in which conspiracy theories can flourish.'

It doesn't take many lobbying scandals to teach the public that elected leaders write laws to suit the highest bidder. From the outside, gatherings of industrial, financial and political bigwigs – the annual World Economic Forum in Davos or the Bilderberg Group conference – resemble flagrant displays of anti-democratic elite collaboration. But a question needs to be raised about the attendees' commitment to secretive plotting if they let the venue and timing of their plots leak into the public domain so often.

The 2008 financial crisis was exceptionally persuasive as a demonstration that wealthy people enjoy immunity from consequence of their wrongdoing. Recognition that banks were too big to fail showed how small national politics had become relative to global capital. The bill for bad judgement exhibited by a financial elite in the City was sent to ordinary tax-paying citizens. That spectacle, coupled with the absence of prosecutions or even punitive economic sanctions for the perpetrators, was a lavish resource supporting the claim that democratic institutions are just a front for financial interests.

That judgement can be true enough to correctly locate a flaw in the system – a weakness that reform and regulation could address – without being *exclusively* true. The existence of corruption doesn't prove that all ministerial power is a sham. The excessive influence of corporate donors doesn't make elections redundant. It can be true that money and greed warp politics without breaking democracy.

It is rational to be wary of corporate power, but that doesn't have to become a populist harangue that calls every profit theft and treats any private sector involvement in public administration as an affront to democracy.

There is a line, not always easy to trace, between scepticism and cynicism; and an arc on which the latter bends round into hypercynicism – the refusal to imagine that politicians can have motives other than venal ones. Cynicism leads to disengagement; hypercynicism is expressed as hyper-engagement – a compulsive attention to detail; a neurotic fixation on hidden processes and obscure events when the banal truth is more likely to be in plain sight.

The hyper-engaged observers are so focused on the intricate operation of political machinery that they overlook the crucial fact that politicians are also, like them, human beings. Their fallibility causes bad things to happen but also makes it likelier that they happen by accident.

That isn't to deny that politicians can be guilty of crimes, negligence and, sometimes, conspiracies. Part of retaining confidence in democracy is retaining awareness of its vulnerabilities, which entails sometimes extending the benefit of the doubt to politicians and also knowing when to withdraw it. That is easier when you think of them as human, which is also easier when you meet them often. But anyone who is intimate enough with power to believe that some of the people exercising it are doing their best with good intentions is a discredited witness in the eyes of those who scan from afar looking for proof that it is all callous corruption.

I have been invited to private dinners with politicians and business leaders in corporate boardrooms. I have attended conferences, including events held in stately homes where the evening dress-code is black tie and the guest list includes ministers, opposition MPs, corporate lobbyists and chief executives. These gigs are usually conducted off the record or under the Chatham House rule, which allows use of the gist of what is said but not reporting of who said it. Lurking on the periphery of that august company, I am usually struck by a disparity between the conversation in the room and the sinister aspect that a fictionalized account of the gathering could acquire. The participants nearly always fret about public opinion and their own impotence in shifting it.

I remember one dinner on the top floor of the Shell Centre in London, hosted by a pro-European think tank, attended by representatives from big business and the City, a couple of fellow journalists, some civil servants, government advisers and

MPs. David Cameron had announced his ambition to hold a referendum on EU membership, but no date was set. The thrust of the conversation was that Brexit would be a terrible idea, and almost certainly wouldn't happen. There was consensus also that free movement of people was a good thing and that more people needed persuading of that fact. I remember coming away from the dinner with a dark sense of foreboding. If it was only bankers and politicians in favour of migration from EU countries and they were afraid to make the case in public, the campaign to leave was shooting at an open goal.

But also, I couldn't help picturing us all in frock coats and stovepipe hats – a scene from some 1930s caricature of a capitalist cabal, or an illustration from *The Protocols of the Elders of Zion*. I don't think I was the only person with Jewish heritage in the room either. I imagined a disappointed Lidia Sergeevna tutting. But we're the *good* ones, I might have explained.

Yes, we were doing exactly what conspiracy theorists would imagine us doing just by being in the room together. But two important details made it not a conspiracy. No one present could agree what had to be done, and none of us had the faintest idea how to achieve the outcome we wanted.

Part Three

REVOLUTION

CHAPTER 10

THE BROKEN PENDULUM

'What happens if I press this button?'

'I wouldn't . . .'

'Oh.'

'What happened?'

'A sign lit up, saying "Please do not press this button again."'

Douglas Adams

(i) Meshugas

A portion of everyone's politics is inherited. We absorb the influence of our parents or rebel against it, in which case the legacy is still there, but inverted. In some families, the habit of voting for a particular party is passed down for preservation like an heirloom. Others acquire no fixed allegiance, but heritable instincts and aversions. From my parents, I received a horror of *meshugas*.

The word is Yiddish and has no direct English counterpart. It is commonly translated as craziness, but encompasses mania, stupidity, wildness, irrationality, intemperance, pointless persistence and general disorderliness in life and mind. It can apply to a person, a situation, a country.

Meshugas is an accusation that says as much about the accuser's state of mind as it does about the offence. It speaks of exasperation tinged with weary fatalism. The complaint against the *meshuggener* (the crazy person) is that their *meshugas* is intrusive, up in your face, inescapable. It won't leave you in peace. It cold-calls you in the middle of the day and wags a hectoring finger at you from the night-time news.

Fear of *meshugas* is a common feature in the first-generation-immigrant psyche, and not just among Jews. People who have crossed continents to start a new life often want to be un-molested by politics, especially if the family story contains recent experience of traumatic upheaval. The opposite can also be true. Exile has been the making of many radicals. But I grew up with a bias for moderation and an ingrained suspicion of politicians who roused rabbles and thumped tubs – the ones with a *meshuggeh* glint in their eye.

The early eighties were awash with *meshugas*. It put the iron in the Iron Lady and the militancy in Labour's Militant Tendency.

One of the only times I recall my dad being actively engaged in party politics was an afternoon in 1981 when he loaded us into the car and drove across London to a rally of the newly formed Social Democratic Party. We got there late and had to stand at the back. All I could see was a tiny body on the monitor screen of a TV camera obscuring my view of the stage. It was Roy Jenkins, the former Labour Home Secretary, who was one of the SDP's founding 'Gang of Four'. I had never seen a live politician in action before. I understood nothing of what was being said but was impressed that it might be on television.

Constrained by an electoral system that favoured entrenched big parties, the SDP failed to break the Labour–Tory duopoly. It merged with the old Liberals to become the Liberal Democrats, mopping up protest votes, causing the occasional by-election upset and haunting the moderate right of the Labour Party as a cautionary tale. The moral of the story, retold many times in the era of Corbynite *meshugas*, was that forming new parties was a waste of time.*

But the SDP was also briefly popular – leading national opinion polls for a short period after its launch. Novelty value was a factor, but the new party also filled a vacancy. It appealed to middle-ground voters made politically homeless by the polarized choice between rampant Thatcherism and dogmatic socialism. That space was eventually colonized by New Labour.

The middle way that Blair found to electoral triumph was not in the same place as the one the SDP had tried to map in 1981. Four Tory election victories had reshaped the political landscape. But as geometry, the principle was much the same – appealing to people who wanted rid of the Conservatives but were wary of politics that leaned too heavily left.

Not everyone calls it a principle. For people who like their politics unalloyed, the third-way meld was at best a campaign expedient, at worst a pollution of Labour's soul. It worked, though, for a decade. The Blairite riposte to the purists was that winning power by compromising with voters allows a party to enact some of its principles as policy, while keeping them pristine in opposition helps no one.

---

* That judgement was twice vindicated. First by the fate of Change UK, founded in 2019 by pro-European Tory dissidents and anti-Corbyn Labour moderates. It was annihilated in the election later that year. Second by the fact that Labour's moderates did eventually recapture the burned-out shell of their former party.

Political identity is buttressed by fixed beliefs, and winning elections involves some movement with the flow of public opinion. There will always be tension there. It is the defining quandary of the doctrine (or is it a non-doctrine?) called centrism.

The term is slippery, not least because it is so commonly used pejoratively. What it means to be a centrist has become inseparable from the Remain campaign in 2016 and the sense that it had misjudged the national mood, missed fundamental changes in the character of British politics and generally found itself on the wrong side of history. Centrism became an explanation for the failure of the thing it described more than an account of the thing itself.

Brexit was an electoral insurrection against a political and economic status quo. Its opponents were drawn from different parties and disagreed on many things, but they found common cause in wanting to prevent what they saw as a colossal act of national self-sabotage. Every former prime minister, Labour and Tory, was a Remainer, as was the incumbent.

That accord facilitated the Leave campaign's strategy of making EU membership the lightning rod for decades of accumulated grievance about other issues.* Remain was the palace of elite self-satisfaction, Versailles for a liberal *ancien régime* against which Brexit was the revolution.

That image conflated two different definitions of the centre. It was a geographical location at the heart of politics – Westminster; the centre of power – and it was the zone of broad

---

* It didn't help that the word 'remain' was redolent of stasis, complacent satisfaction with things as they are, when 'leave' had the dynamic energy of a stride towards better things. For that reason, the pro-European side had wanted the official designations to be 'in' and 'out'.

ideological consensus that had governed Britain, with some modifications, since Blair's 1997 landslide victory. It was the creed of a political Establishment.

Brexit was also an elite project. But it animated a different segment of the Establishment – the reactionary part that had felt rudely brushed aside in the millennial march of metropolitan liberalism. The genius of the Leave campaign was to renew crusty old-school Tory fear of cultural obsolescence with a twenty-first-century populist message for anyone who was disoriented by globalization and felt they had not been adequately consulted on the social changes it brought.

Brexit took a commonplace frustration at the remoteness of power and harnessed it to a rarefied topic that had previously exercised only schismatic Tory malcontents and outliers on the hard-right fringe.

The result was a revolution that, to the consternation of its opponents, was authentic and bogus at the same time. It was a bona fide backlash against elite complacency and a heist – a smash-and-grab raid on power by a rival gang within the elite. It was executed by deft political ju-jitsu. Brexiteers identified the greatest strength of the Remain cause – the fact that it was endorsed by almost everyone who knew anything about sound government, trade economics and international diplomacy – and turned it into a weakness.

Credentials that would once have imbued a political message with credibility were used to deplete its authenticity. Michael Gove expressed the point neatly in an interview in June 2016: 'I think the people in this country have had enough of experts from organizations with acronyms saying that they know what is best and getting it consistently wrong.'*

It was a revolt against established authority, but not an overthrow of elite political power, which passed smoothly from one pair of Conservative hands to another. To the extent that Brexit effected regime change, it happened within the ranks of the same party that had ruled Britain for most of the previous 100 years. But it was a storming of citadels held by self-styled cultural and cognitive elites. It was an invitation to get one over on the smug know-it-all types whose lofty urbanity was European in the sense that it carried a whiff of continental hauteur.

The Establishment to be overthrown could thus be construed as any institution that weighed evidence in its assessment of the case for leaving the EU. That damned universities, the BBC, the civil service, the Bank of England, the Institute for Fiscal Studies, the Confederation of British Industry, the Institute of Directors, most trade unions and large numbers of people in both Houses of Parliament. (Not covered by that definition of the Establishment were half of David Cameron's cabinet, scores of Tory MPs, the proprietors of the *Daily Mail*, the *Daily Express*, *The Sun* and the *Telegraph*, and the wealthy donors who financed the Leave campaign.)

---

* As with Theresa May's 'citizens of nowhere' line, Gove's 'had enough of experts' comment became notorious shorn of its contextualizing follow-on clauses. It is marginally less sinister in the fuller version, but the implication is not that different to the one commonly attributed to it. A list of such quotes might include Thatcher claiming there was no such thing as society. Fuller quote: 'Who is society? There is no such thing! There are individual men and women and there are families and no government can do anything except through people and people look to themselves first.' Also, Peter Mandelson saying New Labour was intensely relaxed about people getting filthy rich – 'as long as they pay their taxes'. The subordinate clauses blunt the edge of the one that was immortalized, but folk memory has correctly preserved the gist.

Brexit did not eliminate the old left–right distinction from British politics, but it did revolutionize the geometry, with Remain and Leave as opposite poles and badges of cultural identity.

There was no middle way between being in or out of the EU. The issue was irreducibly binary. Attempts at compromise failed because the hard-line Eurosceptics saw incremental models of Brexit as pointless facsimiles of EU membership, or worse. Remainers agreed. If leaving was understood as a principled rupture to achieve national redemption, there could be no half-measures. And pro-Europeans measured separation from Britain's neighbours in degrees of damage that could only be avoided by calling the whole thing off.

If a centrist was someone who supported EU membership, they ceased to be in the centre after the referendum, since by definition they were on one side of a partisan divide. In the 2019 general election, a centrist was someone (like me) who hated to see Boris Johnson in Downing Street and winced at the thought of Jeremy Corbyn being there instead. Those symmetrical repulsions landed a voter in the middle of nowhere. The centre was neither a coherent ideological position nor a place where elections were won.

But it was still a sanctuary from the *meshugas* that became the normal state of politics after Brexit.

(ii) Boom and bust

The collapse of the centre felt sudden for those of us who were standing on it, but that is because we hadn't been paying attention to shifting ground beneath our feet. The place we were standing might not have been so central after all. The centre moves. It has shifted rightwards through most of my lifetime.

In the early 1980s, Thatcherism was a radical new doctrine with opponents still on the 'wet' side of the Tory cabinet. By the mid nineties, it was the foundation of the UK economy. It made sense for Blair to steer between pro-market conservatism and state-managed socialism. The centrist view at that time held that Thatcher's economics had delivered national prosperity but meanly shared, with a callous sink-or-swim social policy. The left was thought charitable but inept, contaminated by memories of the dysfunctional late seventies: stagnation, inflation, industrial strife, decline.

Those presumptions seemed reliable enough to form the basis of economic orthodoxy and political strategy through the Great Moderation (as described in Chapter 3). There was no need for recalibration when the economy was growing, which it did, uninterrupted, for 16 years.

Then the music stopped.

I first understood what it meant for boom to go bust one evening in September 2008. It was an editorial conference at the *Observer*. Banks were not lending to each other. The City of London was mired in toxic debt and frozen in panic. A colleague who was well connected with the government briefed us on what he had just heard from the Treasury. He was agitated. However bad we thought things were looking, he told us, they were worse. Britain was days, or more likely hours away from ATM machines not working; panic-buying, pandemonium.

I went straight from that meeting to drinks with friends, but I couldn't re-engage with the world around me. The booming London nightlife was as raucous as ever. And all I could think, weaving through the throng, was how the people all around me were oblivious. I felt as if I had just come from a NASA briefing about a meteor on a collision course with earth, and all these people were partying like they had no idea.

What followed was as much a crisis of trust as economics. Hardly anyone had seen the disaster coming. Gordon Brown had boasted that the cycle of boom and bust was eliminated. The market – unimpeachable authority on the efficient allocation of resources for a successful economy – had failed. This was partly what Gove meant a decade later in Brexit debates, or rather the suspicion he was able to mobilize cynically when he said that people had heard enough from so-called economic 'experts'.

The radioactive meltdown of the financial system in 2007–8 contaminated politics for a long time. National governments had propped up the whole system with state revenue. Voters could think of better uses of their tax money than bail-outs for bankers. It looked as if the villains who had caused the mess in the first place were being rewarded for failure with money diverted from the people who were blameless. It looked that way because that's how it was.

Into the crater blown open by financial calamity landed the bombshell of the 2009 parliamentary expenses scandal. Faith in the probity of Parliament was hollowed out by revelations that many MPs had been gaming the remuneration system to top up their salaries, furnish their second homes and take care of their mortgages. The market was dysfunctional and the authority of the legislature was eviscerated.

That was a dramatic moment in British politics, but in hindsight a less pivotal one than it should have been. Expectation of a vast upheaval, expressed as widespread insistence that there could not possibly be a return to 'business as usual', was followed by government that felt to many people like business as usual.

There were electoral and ideological reasons why crisis begat stasis. The Tories were in the ascendant after their long sojourn in the electoral wilderness but came to the financial crisis primed to misdiagnose its causes and dispense the wrong remedies. They were disinclined by culture and doctrine to find fault with free markets, so they attributed all problems to excessive public spending and borrowing by Gordon Brown. The result was budget austerity that visited the cost of repairing public finances on the people who were most dependent on state services, without an obvious dividend in restored growth.

Labour was theoretically better equipped to offer a critique of post-Thatcherite economics, except they had been the incumbent government, presiding over the failure they wanted to denounce. The political pendulum that might have expressed a natural movement from right to left in response to a capitalist malfunction was broken.

In the 2010 general election, Labour lost but the Tories didn't quite win. Public appetite for something – anything – other than the standard blue and red items on the menu was expressed in a sudden surge of support for the Liberal Democrats, especially after their leader, Nick Clegg, out-performed his rivals in a televised debate. One poll at the height of the ensuing 'Cleggmania' had the Lib Dems in pole position on 34 per cent, ahead of the Tories on 31 per cent and Labour on 26 per cent.

They finished, as usual, in third place, but took enough of a bite from their rivals' share to deliver a hung parliament. Their reward was a coalition government with the Tories and five years of brand annihilation. The Lib Dems had spent the previous decade attacking New Labour from the left. Climbing into bed with Cameron confirmed a long-held view among the Labour faithful that compromise to capture the centre was just a euphemism for prostitution to the Tories.*

A symmetrical resentment was stewing on the right. Cameron's efforts to make his party electable by 'modernization' had been cribbed from the New Labour playbook. The implicit contract that the Tory leader offered to his ideological right wing was a copy-and-paste version of the one Blair had once offered the Labour left – acquiescence to a platform they didn't like in exchange for power. The strategy was to cast Cameron unashamedly as the 'heir to Blair'. But the 2010 result looked nothing like 1997. The right felt cheated.

Coalition government added injury to insult, making fewer ministerial jobs available for Tory MPs who already felt neglected and sometimes despised by their leader. (Cameron's barb about 'loonies, fruitcakes and closet racists' had been aimed at UKIP, but it stuck in plenty of Tories too.) He used cabinet appointments as a signal of commitment to racial diversification and gender equality. That left a lot of mediocre middle-aged white Tory men feeling robbed of their entitle-ment to a ministry. Away from Westminster, the role of general-purpose repository for protest votes, once provided by the Lib Dems, was taken over by UKIP. Nigel Farage seized

---

* In the campaign, Clegg and his MP candidates signed a pledge not to raise student university tuition fees and then broke it before the year was out. He and his party were bywords for betrayal and duplicity for the rest of their term in office.

the vacancy as unofficial leader of the none-of-the-above movement.*

By the end of 2010, the conditions were already in place for 'centrism' to be vilified as the doctrine of unprincipled power grabs, economic stagnation and bloodless technocratic leadership by a caste of slickly presentable posh-sounding men in navy blue suits.

My view of British democracy at this time was still flattered by the comparison with the Potemkin version I had observed in Russia. I was frustrated by the common assertion that the main parties and their leaders were 'all the same', probably because I was professionally obliged to concentrate on their differences. On economic policy, for example, there was a measurable gap between Conservative austerity and Labour's resistance to it. But it required some unpacking of Keynesian economics to make the case.

It was like reporting on a tactical card game being played in a vast arena. If you knew all the rules and stood close enough, you could judge the strengths of different hands and how well the players performed. But for the audience in the back rows, the spectacle was distant and barely comprehensible.

A lack of ideological definition was compounded by the trend of increasing professionalization. Politics had become a technical pursuit, practised by a cadre of thrusting young graduates. They took their apprenticeships as special advisers, and used the contacts thus acquired to wangle safe parliamentary

---

* The policy overlap between UKIP and the Lib Dems was negligible, and there was not vast traffic in voters between them, although it happened more than their diametrically opposed stances on the European question might suggest.

seats, which were secure launch pads for ministerial office. In the 2010–15 parliament, the prime minister, the Chancellor, the leader of the opposition, then Ed Miliband, and the shadow Chancellor, Ed Balls, had all arrived at the top of their respective party pyramids by that route.

Disappointment with the narrow menu of options was felt equally by party activists and disengaged voters, although they had different views of what should change. The Tory right had sat through 13 years of Labour government and was itching for redress. But the stalwart socialist left had also felt the Blair and Brown years as a time of banishment.

Each end of the spectrum had a comforting story to tell itself about historical forces moving in its direction. For the right, the financial crisis proved the adage that Labour always runs out of other people's money. For the left, it was the death throes of a free-market capitalist model. The overarching feeling of stasis matched the characterization of an interregnum, as defined by the Marxist philosopher Antonio Gramsci. In conditions where 'the old is dying and the new cannot be born', he wrote, 'a great variety of morbid symptoms appear'.

Everyone thought they were owed a swing of the pendulum.

Seismic activity in Scottish politics gave some advance warning of changes that would soon also be felt at Westminster, but England, typically, wasn't listening. The 2014 independence vote brought a surge in participation, lifting turnout to 85 per cent – 20 points higher than it had been in the general election four years earlier. When people believed their vote would count for something, and the ballot paper posed a drastic enough question, they felt compelled to answer.

Nationalism offered a way for Scottish voters to escape the

Labour–Tory duopoly – a direction for politics to swing when the conventional left–right pendulum was broken. Although the Yes campaign for Scottish independence lost the referendum, it entrenched a new political alignment and accelerated the decay of old allegiances. In the UK general election of 2010, the SNP had won 6 of the 59 available seats in Scotland. In 2015, they took 56, including seats that had been solidly Labour for generations.

It was a collapse that prefigured the fall of the so-called 'red wall' to Boris Johnson four years later. Scottish voters in traditionally Labour-held, working-class heartland seats had come to feel neglected, and culturally remote from the Westminster party. Many were also deeply allergic to the idea of ever putting a cross in the box next to a Tory candidate's name. Nationalism gave them the option of casting off a hereditary Labour allegiance without activating the Tory-hating antibodies in their political bloodstream. It would take another referendum, a few more years of stagnant interregnum, the vote-repelling properties of Jeremy Corbyn, and Boris Johnson's magnetism to swing England's Labour heartlands.

David Cameron took a lesson from the Scottish independence vote, but the wrong one. He saw that nationalism had been beaten by arguments based on brute economic logic.* The case for independence had been countered with hard-headed rational rebuttals about the practical implications of separation

---

* Also, in 2015, Cameron had won the majority that had eluded the Tories five years earlier. It gave him an inflated sense of his powers of persuasion. He thought he could then ride the pendulum all the way to victory in a European referendum that he had only signed up to as a sop to keep the anti-Brussels fanatics in his party quiet.

from England; what it would mean in terms of security, prosperity and stability. It was too much of a gamble. That strategy – 'Project Fear' – was tweaked and remodelled as the case for Britain staying in the EU.

It didn't work. Some of the reasons why were examined in Part One. The referendum gave shape to cultural divisions and exposed fault lines that ran deeper than sympathy for the European project. The emotional charge that might have energized the Remain cause was mostly unleashed by the shock of defeat, by which point Leave had the democratic high ground.

The 2019 general election result then reinforced the idea that Brexit had been all about the sudden activation of political consciousness in former Labour heartlands. Those were the same 'red wall' seats that gave Boris Johnson his majority. Hindsight merged a parliamentary landslide with a narrowly won plebiscite and branded both as phases of the same revolt by voters who felt 'left behind' by globalization.

It is a resonant cultural story, true up to a point but easily over-mythologized.

The bedrock of the Leave vote was people who had voted for David Cameron in 2015. If they had backed him on the referendum too, Britain would still be a member of the EU, regardless of what happened in Workington or Sunderland. The genius of the pro-Brexit campaign was to find a point of alignment between affluent southern Tories and Labour's crumbling electoral bedrock.

The Leave campaign also got an edge by mobilizing formerly apathetic voters; people who had become chronically disengaged. Liz Kendall, a Labour MP, described the campaign in terms of a big red button marked 'Brexit'. Voters didn't necessarily know what it would involve, but they understood that the prime minister and a lot of other politicians were afraid of it. Also, this wasn't an ordinary election, where nothing really changed. If the button was pressed, everything would be shaken up and wouldn't go back to the way it was before. Then the Remainers came along and said: 'Please don't press the button.' Kendall's explanation for the result: 'What the hell else did we think they were going to do?'

The day after the referendum, one senior figure in the Remain campaign told me: 'I knew we'd lost when someone at a polling station asked me how it all worked. He looked a bit lost. He'd clearly never voted in his life. He turned to me and said, "Where do I go for the Leave?"' Turnout in the EU referendum was 72 per cent, compared to 66 per cent in the 2015 general election. (The low point in recent decades was 59 per cent in 2001, when Tony Blair was in his pomp and the Tories were in the wilderness.)

There was also something compelling about the invitation to deliver change through a mechanism that was not just another election. It was a different, stronger, saltier flavour of democracy. The problem was that it then left the other kind – the fiddly business of parliamentary representation – seeming insipid and inconsequential.

Former Labour voters are more analysed in the composition of the Brexit vote because their choice described a more profound cultural realignment than the decision of Tory Leavers. It is hard to know how much of that voter migration was a function of the immediate crisis and how much was the harvest of disillusionment sown over decades. Johnson's slogan 'Get

Brexit Done' had the potent subtext 'Make Them Stop', in which *they* were all the bickering, point-scoring, troublesome politicians from whose ranks he artfully distinguished himself.

But before Brexit was even on the radar, Labour MPs were warning that their support had become threadbare. It was a ghost of the former allegiance – literally so, to the extent that many people on the doorstep told canvassers that they only backed the party for fear that their dead parents would turn in their graves if they ever thought their children were voting Tory.

The New Labour years, when budgets were bulging, had postponed this reckoning. Blair and Brown addressed financial deprivation in places that had been hollowed out by industrial decline in the Thatcher years. Public services were expanded, schools and hospitals were refurbished, shiny new libraries and children's centres appeared. Cash transfers gave economic life support but did not repair the loss of local esteem – the feeling of marginalization, of being *culturally* left behind as London soared ahead as the national centre of political and economic gravity.

The choice of Jeremy Corbyn as Labour leader in 2015 didn't solve that problem, despite his supporters' conviction that weakness in the party's bones was caused by a deficiency of vitamin socialism. The misdiagnosis was seductive. There was evidence that could be construed to make the case in soaring membership, rallies that had the energy of revivalist churches, and the 2017 general election, where Corbyn's support surged, confounding Westminster expectation. Theresa May had only called the election because she was so confident of trouncing him. But Labour still lost, and the subsequent years of Brexit impasse exposed the gulf between the party's activist base and the voters they needed to win a general election.

The ideological vanguard of Corbynism was led by university-educated radicals, many of whom were too young to remember the Cold War, and geezers wearing hammer-and-sickle lapel badges who thought the wrong side had won. That project was never going to appeal to people who had voted for Brexit because they were angry about uncontrolled immigration and who saw in Corbyn a man quick to defend Britain's overseas enemies and tongue-tied when the national anthem played.

On the European question, Corbyn was sceptical on anti-capitalist grounds – as a project too amenable to corporate interests.* He was coaxed into desultory endorsement of the Remain cause because that was where the overwhelming majority of Labour members wanted him to be. Once the result was in, he assumed a position of peevish detachment from Brexit. He neither pressed for its completion nor agitated for annulment. He drummed his fingers on the sidelines of the national debate, tutting resentfully because the wrong revolution had barged the queue to make history when it was meant to be his turn.†

---

* This was the reason why the socialist left opposed Britain's EEC accession in the 1970s. Objection to that position when it became Labour policy in the early 1980s was a cause of the schism that created the pro-European SDP.

† Corbyn's supporters argue that Labour's strong performance in the 2017 general election proved there was more of an appetite for radical-left policies than Conservatives and centrists had anticipated. Labour's manifesto had wider appeal than its leader. The result of that ballot is hard to unpick because Theresa May fought a self-sabotaging campaign and the Labour vote share was a confused alliance of people who supported the party *because* of Corbyn and those who carried on voting for their old party *in spite of* its leader. There was enough ambiguity for partisans of every position to persuade themselves that they had been right all along.

(iii) Centre folded

There was a counter-revolution of sorts. Organized under the banner of the 'People's Vote' campaign for a referendum rematch, it succeeded in radicalizing Remainer feeling but failed to change Leavers' minds.

The battle got bogged down in parliamentary procedure. Remainers kept winning tactical skirmishes over constitutional foothills; the Leavers held fast to the democratic heights of the argument – that Brexit had to be done because a majority had voted for it. Pro-Europeans were still litigating the wisdom of ending Britain's strategic and economic alliances and fretting about the moral character of a nationalist enterprise. The Brexiteers simply asked what part of Leave had been so hard to understand the first time?

In that climate, 'centrism' became a byword for abject political failure. It was a target for the Corbynite left and the Brexiteer right alike. We could be lumped together with all the unloved Establishment institutions – pre-referendum party elites; the City of London; big business. We were also politically destitute, a ragged itinerant bunch, represented in Parliament by quitters and loners – Blairite Labour MPs sulking in Corbyn's shadow; the vestiges of pro-European Toryism; Lib Dems. Centrists were a stale crust of a coalition with no policy platform, no leadership, and nothing much to say about the future, except that it should look more like the recent past.

The core problem for centrism was ambiguity on whether it was meant to describe an ideological position or an electoral tactic. The generous view configures it as principled avoidance of extreme dogmas, left and right. In a harsher light it looks like a recipe for jettisoning any principle for its opposite if that is the more efficient route to power. That distinction mattered less when centrists were winning. It could be argued that half an ideal enacted in government was better than a whole one nursed in impotent opposition. But if centrism wasn't even a great electoral strategy, then really, what was the point?

In 2017, Giles Fraser, a pro-Brexit Corbyn supporter, wrote a column in the *Guardian* under the headline 'Rejoice! Centrism in British Politics is Dead and Big Ideas are Back'. His autopsy included this verdict:

> Unlike those who want to change the world, the defining feature of centrists is not a belief in any particular kind of political philosophy but simply a supreme confidence in their ability to run things. They gaze out on to the messy political fray with a superior disdain, ready to step in and adjudicate some sensible compromise. Politics is a management exercise led by suitably educated professionals.

Two years later, during the Tory leadership contest that would install Boris Johnson in Downing Street, Matthew Lesh, of the libertarian Adam Smith Institute, punched the same bruise in the *Daily Telegraph*. Dismissing the 'vacuous centrism' of Rory Stewart, the Tory moderates' candidate, Lesh declared:

> In practice, those who attempt to sit at the 'centre point' will inevitably be thrown around in the wind. This is because the centre moves at different times and places, what is reasonable in one context is not in another, therefore if you just merely

try to aim for the centre you will inevitably end up deeply inconsistent and at the whims of others who do stand for something.

Enough of that critique was true to be wounding – the part where centrism had shrivelled into a complaint about the un-fitness of Corbyn and Johnson for high office. But the complaint had solid foundations, as events quickly demonstrated. The centrists could be most of the things their critics denigrated them for, while still correct in their judgement that Brexit was a bad idea and in their repugnance at the options on the 2019 ballot paper.

What that election said about Britain and its enthusiasm for Brexit as a revolution is less clear-cut than was claimed by Johnson and the MPs who followed in his slipstream. There was no serious debate about the actual consequences of leaving the EU under the terms on offer (or any terms). Radicals of left and right also had common incentives to cast the events of the previous years as proof that centrist moderation was an obsolete creed.

Liberal Britain experienced a spasm of self-pity tinged with self-loathing as it contemplated the effects of its complacency over the previous decades. That guilt-ridden capitulation, justified in some respects, awarded the Brexiteers a bonus moral victory. It left unchallenged their claim to be tribunes of the people in opposition to a distant and haughty elite.

That vulnerability has a lot in common with a weakness of the American left in the years preceding Donald Trump's capture of the White House. One lucid account of it was published in April 2016, in an essay for *Vox* magazine by

Emmett Rensin, under the title 'The Smug Style in American Liberalism'.*

Rensin's critique was that college-educated white-collar liberals were prone to supercilious frustration with the opinions and manners of the working-class voters who had for years delivered battleground states for the Democratic Party. That attitude had been kept in check by various forces – trade union links and electoral pragmatism among them. Then the white working class drifted away, a bit under Nixon, a lot under Reagan. Bill Clinton and Barack Obama failed to reverse the trend. Liberalism became unbalanced. A smug style took over, explaining every setback as a problem of false consciousness and intellectual backwardness. As Rensin's caustic précis of the liberal view put it: 'The trouble is that stupid hicks don't know what's good for them. They're getting conned by right-wingers and tent revivalists until they believe all the lies that've made them so wrong. They don't know any better. That's why they're *voting against their own self-interest.*' With a small adjustment of idiom and accent, that could sound like dismay on the British liberal left at working-class support for Brexit and Boris Johnson in 2019.

This is the part of the centrist defeat that I found hardest to navigate. I saw contradictory things that were simultaneously true: Brexit sprang from real grievance and nationalist fiction; it was richly symbolic and a cheap scam; it was procured by a campaign of lies that gave a democratic voice to people who had felt unheard for a generation; it signalled the bankruptcy

---

* That was an allusion to Richard Hofstadter's seminal 1964 essay for *Harper's* on 'The Paranoid Style in American Politics', which located McCarthyism in a longer tradition of witch-hunting and irrational superstition.

of centrist politics but the centrist complaint about it was not all wrong.

No less infuriating: a reservoir of potential energy for radical reform to the way Britain is governed was squandered on a cause that only aggravated the demand for change. Almost as tragic, the Labour opposition had a parallel misspent revolution of its own, marrying an idealistic young generation off to Corbyn and desiccated left-fogeyism.

The revolution was real. The revolution was phoney. Politics was stuck and also moving at speed; racing into crisis and mired in stasis. The pendulum was swinging wildly, while by-passing the centre ground. Much of the ensuing volatility, the state of permacrisis that consumed British democracy after the referendum, was an expression of those contradictions. Brexit came to mean entirely different things, confusingly denoted by the same word. It was a myth of national liberation and a technical job of dismantling the country's long-established trade and diplomatic relationships.

When the Conservatives found themselves confounded by the practical task in hand (which happened often) they took refuge in fantasy. The various changes of prime minister since 2016 have all had their specific circumstances and proximate causes, but they also described the constant attrition of a Conservative party dosing itself with ideology and hurling itself at a brick wall of reality. In a word: *meshugas*.

CHAPTER 11

INSIDE OUT

You cannot hope to bribe or twist,
Thank God! the British journalist.
But, seeing what the man will do
unbribed, there's no occasion to.

Humbert Wolfe

(i) The long spoon

Nigel Farage ordered another gin and tonic, draining the one he had started before I arrived. It was around noon on a damp English summer day. We were in the restaurant attached to Brown's Hotel, a venue of medium grandeur by Mayfair standards, neither subtle nor flamboyant, occupying what used to be a row of white stucco-fronted Georgian townhouses.

This was to be lunch in the old-fashioned Fleet Street sense of the word; what a certain generation of journalist called a 'proper lunch', after which only a veteran of that era, having developed a formidable tolerance for alcohol, would be capable of filing copy later in the afternoon. A rookie would hardly see the typewriter.

An older colleague once advised me to take regular toilet

breaks to make notes about conversations of which my memory might end up patchy. That wasn't necessary with Farage, because he took such frequent cigarette breaks, not just between courses but between mouthfuls of food within courses.

This was 2013, and I was political editor at the *New Statesman* magazine. It was not the first time I had met Farage, but it was the only time we sat down together. The third person at the table was Stuart Wheeler, a former Tory financier who had switched his allegiance and his munificence to UKIP. I had met Wheeler at a dinner hosted by a right-wing think tank that had also benefited from his political philanthropy. My attendance at the dinner was part of a mercenary networking campaign, undertaken to rebalance a contacts book that was skewed liberal and left. The Tories were in government and looked likely to stay there. I needed to spend more time chewing the cud with people from the other side, the people who were setting the news agenda, people like Farage.

I saw two problems with this plan. First, I would rather chew wasps. Second, it wasn't obvious why the contacts I wanted to cultivate would want to spend any time with me. The *New Statesman* was in those days seen as a socialist trade mag; a niche publication that right-wingers treated as an exotic and inhospitable part of the media ecosystem. The editor had asked me to make them feel more welcome.

Over a proper lunch, I was capable of sounding ecumenical and striking up a rapport with people whose politics I disliked. The challenge was doing it without hating myself. The trick was to find the small portion of someone's opinion that I could agree with – usually there was something – and express it back to them in a way that made them think I was amenable to hearing more. I could dispatch cagey conversational ambassadors to open diplomatic relations across ideological divides. Also, everyone in Westminster loves to gossip. The trade in that commodity crosses even the most hostile party lines.

By that method I had persuaded Wheeler to set up lunch with Farage. The UKIP leader was mostly interested in my perspective on Labour – a realm to which he had limited access. In exchange, he had some insights to share about the most Eurosceptic faction of the Tory party and some candour about the deficiencies of his own party – the difficulty in recruiting reliable parliamentary candidates, which I understood to mean people who were fluent in the idiom of respectable dudgeon, lamenting the state of Britain without blundering into flagrant bigotry. Or, at the very least, people who didn't post pictures of themselves giving Nazi salutes on social media.

That is generally what is meant in politics by the verb *to lunch* – to negotiate a tactical exchange of indiscretions. By a campaign of lunching, I was learning to be an insider, or to pose as one at least. I was well aware of how much better connected other people were, and how tenuous my connection was to the loop that connected real insiders. But almost everyone in Westminster has some insecurity about their proximity to the loop. Backbench MPs feel cut out of it because they are not in government offices; junior ministers feel excluded from cabinet; cabinet ministers crave more access to No. 10; people inside No. 10 want more time with the prime minister. Almost everyone feels they are on the wrong side of a closing door much of the time. And then prime ministers get paranoid that the world outside their own office is all plots and intrigues against them.

A lot of political journalism is about gaming that insecurity, trading information, trying to verify gossip, hearing half a story and finagling the other half out of someone who wants your half. I came to enjoy it, but never got very good at it. Also, compulsively monitoring the action inside Westminster often meant turning my back on the world outside and wilfully forgetting that most people, most of the time, don't have the time or inclination to follow events in that much detail.

What insiders call politics and what most people think of when they use that word are not the same. Or rather, they describe the same set of activities, using the same word, but imbued with divergent assumptions about what motivates the actors, to what extent they are a caste apart from the rest, how much it is worth caring about them, which of them is to be trusted.

Journalism is supposed to bridge the gap. The wider the distance, the greater the level of public mistrust, the harder it is for the journalist to report on a political class without becoming a member and so compromising their credentials as a dependable source.

When I consider the time I spent loitering in the ante-chambers of government, I can apply two interpretations.

Through the darkest glass, I see complacency and an amoral complicity with power. I could tell myself I was part of a noble enterprise, lubricating the flow of information outward to the wider world, holding the mighty to account wielding only the humble pen. But I also just liked knowing more about what was going on in the corridors of power than people who didn't have special passes to wander them. The theory of the Fourth Estate – the quasi-constitutional function of the media as a pillar of democracy – was a patina of ethical purpose on what was essentially sport for political nerds. Apply that lens in the harshest light and you find traces of what Stanley Baldwin once bemoaned as 'power without responsibility – the prerogative of the harlot throughout the ages'.

But Baldwin was talking about media proprietors. A few boozy lunches with crapulous nationalists hardly makes me a Viscount Rothermere or Rupert Murdoch. I was getting to know political players to pass any insight thus gleaned on to others so they could make up their own minds. That is the kinder lens that projects my insider insinuations as an infiltration, a mission on behalf of the ultimate boss – the reader.

'Remember, they're not your friends,' a veteran American reporter once told me about contacts made in the line of duty. 'They're your prey.' I was never very good at that side of things – the blood sport of scoop-hunting. I was shy of confrontation. I didn't like making enemies and was too keen to make conversations flow. My technique of cagey diplomacy yielded a bunch of contacts, from whom I learned a lot about how politics works, but it didn't often get the story that made the next day's front page.

Then the world I knew began to unravel, or more accurately, the political milieu to which I had become accustomed fell apart. I was left wondering whether I hadn't become one of those birds that subsists on morsels picked from the teeth of a yawning crocodile. You get what you need at the cost of providing oral hygiene to a carnivorous reptile. As Farage's political orbit took in ever more fascistic circles – cosying up to far-right parties elsewhere in Europe and playing warm-up man to the crowds at Donald Trump rallies – I was ashamed to have treated him as just another character on the Westminster stage, breaking bread with him and charging it on expenses.

An old proverb recommends that anyone supping with the devil should carry a long spoon. It has always sounded impractical to me. Once the choice has been made to dine in evil company, the dimensions of the cutlery aren't going to make a difference, except to the number of spillages. The choice is to sup or not to sup; you can guess what goes on in the devil's head or you can ask him. Hugo Young, one of the all-time great political columnists, put it succinctly in the preface to an anthology of his work titled *Supping with the Devils*. 'We need to have relations with them. They own the truths we think we're reporting.' That doesn't oblige us to believe what we are told.

Something still rankles with me about that Farage lunch, and I don't think it is only guilt at having put on a cordial show for a man whose politics repel me. I would feel more embarrassed by that if I had gone easier on him and his party in print to facilitate further access. But I never pretended to think they were anything other than a menace. It is not my hypocrisy that burns after all these years, but his.

I don't mind owning up to the myopia of the insider – focusing always on the room where a bit of present drama is unfolding and forgetting to scan the horizon for signs of history on the move. But I don't accept the warped political geometry that narrates that period as if the inside was a realm governed exclusively by centrists and Remainers, with Euro-sceptics and nationalists on the outside, with the people.

I can understand the frustration of voters hundreds of miles from Westminster who saw the appeal in Brexit on the terms that it was sold to them. I can admit my contribution to a long collective complacency that let the pressure build up sufficiently to make an act of rebellious release feel so necessary. But it boiled my blood when the impeccably credentialled professional politicians who led that revolution excused themselves from belonging to the Establishment so they might claim to be overthrowing it.

But that was the power of Brexit ju-jitsu – the move that defined the losing side as the authors of their own defeat, punished for elite detachment from the will of the people. Lying winded on the mat, I was supposed to believe that the shoulder over which I had just been thrown was in fact mine.

(ii) Join the club

If I had been native to the elite, I might not have felt like an imposter when I joined the parliamentary press lobby. I was allowed to be there, having just taken possession of my security pass, but permission to be on the premises did not dispel the uneasy feeling of trespass. I kept expecting one of the many police officers or parliamentary officials to escort me from the building. It didn't help that the first time I tried to enter the journalists' gallery of the Commons chamber itself, my path was blocked by a man in tights and a frock coat who steered me firmly but politely back through the heavy wooden doors – half teacher, half bouncer – and explained that there was no admittance without a tie.

This is not a hard-luck story of ostracism, nor a claim to have hit any glass or class ceilings on the way to Westminster. Being white, male and an Oxford graduate is hardly the profile of a plucky outsider breaching the walls of institutional prejudice.

I arrived in Oxford in 1992 largely clueless about the university's reputation for anything other than academic excellence. I read *Brideshead Revisited* in the summer after my A levels, but thought it described only the past. I was surprised to meet so many fellow undergraduates who seemed to have stepped from the pages of Evelyn Waugh.

I was surprised, too, by the number of formal occasions where gowns and mortar boards were obligatory. At one such occasion in my first week, I was sarcastically congratulated for wearing a suit that apparently made me look like a used-car salesman (it was a double-breasted bottle-green number from Marks & Spencer). I was no less surprised when a posh young man, one of many old Etonians about the place, described my north London accent as 'cockney',* suggesting that he had never met anyone from lands east of Berkshire.

As Simon Kuper has written in *Chums*, his book about the phenomenal influence of Oxford on British politics, one of the university's most prolific achievements is recruiting people who aren't posh and grooming them to be adjuncts to the apparatus where the poshest thrive. At Oxford, we were 'trained to feel at ease in establishment settings'. But we were also aware that those settings were not laid on for our benefit.

I was loosely interested in politics but had never given any thought to the question of how people actually become politicians. When I first received my offer of a place at the university, the letter came with an application form to join

---

* The absurdity of this appellation should be immediately obvious to anyone who has heard me speak. I sound posher now, after my Oxford training, than I did when I arrived there. But I was not by any stretch of the imagination cockney.

something called the Oxford Union Society. The bumf didn't explain what it was, only that it cost in the region of £100 to join. The form went straight into the bin. Even when I became aware that there was such a thing as a 'union hack', and that it meant candidacy in some kind of election, I didn't understand to what end they were campaigning. After I left Oxford, I learned that the Union is a debating club that styles itself as a junior House of Commons and a test bed for the rhetorical talents of future prime ministers.

I was at the same college at the same time as Liz Truss, but remember very little about her. We studied different things and moved with different crowds. I was too young to have overlapped with David Cameron, George Osborne and Boris Johnson, and was unaware of the Bullingdon Club – the not-very-secret dining society for aristocratic delinquents. A notorious 'Buller' drunken escapade involved breaking windows and trashing restaurants for no other reason than to demonstrate how wanton vandalism has no consequence to the perpetrator whose social safety-net is woven from inherited wealth.

I was certainly aware of the type of person who was recruited to clubs like that. They were hard to miss. There was a style of bellowing arrogance, coupled with menacing bonhomie, in the young men – always men – who seemed to take up more space than anyone else in the room. The force field of their egos extended several inches in every direction around their bodies.

These young men seemed not only to have been fed from an early age on something that gave them the physical bulk required for rugby and rowing, but to have been immersed at birth in some mythic river that covered them with a gloss of impregnable entitlement. Exposure to that subculture in Oxford had a lasting impact on me. It was not necessarily envy or resentment (although those were definitely present in my initial reactions), but an exaggerated and enduring sense of the difference between my own bog-standard middle-class privileges, which came with some ballast of guilt, and the ferocious confidence of England's born-to-rule caste. Their lack of self-doubt was a superpower. It vaporized obstacles on the path to ambition's fulfilment. This is one of the more footling differentiations of the infinitely intricate British class system. But it exists enough that I retained for too long an exaggerated sense of my own separateness from the Establishment. It meant that, years later when I had been fully naturalized as a denizen of Westminster, I was slow to grasp the extent to which insiders, with me in their number, all looked and sounded the same from the outside.

I was no better at appreciating how blurred the difference between journalists and politicians had become, viewed from a distance. Seen close up, the relationship looked mostly adversarial, notwithstanding any boozy commerce in gossip.

Part of the confusion arises from the informal codes of the lobby – the cadre of specially accredited journalists who, among other privileges, attend the daily Downing Street press briefings with the prime minister's official spokesperson.

The term refers to the Members' Lobby, immediately outside the Commons chamber, where traditionally journalists buttonhole MPs on their way in and out of debates. The understanding is that information thus gleaned can be used but not attributed, and nothing that happens in the lobby itself can be reported. (There are finer points of protocol, but that is the gist.)

The lobby system comes in for a lot of criticism: for its historic dominance by white men; for quasi-Masonic secrecy; for cultivating a herd mentality; for being an information cartel that has a vested interest in protecting the Establishment, offering tacit protection in exchange for access; for being too easily seduced by colourful personalities and obsessed with tittle-tattle; for parochialism and cynicism; for allowing itself to be manipulated by crafty spin doctors; for flagrant partisanship and excessive cosiness with contacts.

There is truth in all of those charges, although the lobby also has a record of tenacious pursuit of wrongdoing and has collectively fallen out with every incumbent government in modern times, which suggests it is not entirely prone to capture. As with so much of the British way of doing democracy, the line between cultural foible, clubbability and corruption is not always easy to draw.

There are journalists who become stenographers and activists on behalf of parties and prime ministers, although in my experience, that level of partisanship is not the norm. A trickier problem is the revolving door that operates between the lobby and the ranks of political special advisers (spads). The prime minister's director of communications is often a former political editor, who will bring a legacy of lobby comradeships to the job. With supposed antagonists drawn from such a narrow gene pool, it is easy to breed a conviviality that is not conducive to rigorous press scrutiny of government.

The competitive impulse to get a scoop and the bloodthirstiness in pursuit of a wounded government are countervailing forces, pulling against both complicity and collegiality. The idea that lazy hacks are spoon-fed instruction on what to write is rejected by every spokesman who has had their spoon rejected and its contents spat out.

But the perception that British political journalists serve power instead of holding it to account has formed for a reason. Individual reporters on the *Daily Mail* or *The Sun* might aspire to independence, but unhinged partisanship is the corporate ethos for much of Fleet Street. Even the part that is hinged mostly swings to the right. When the Tory press guns for Conservative prime ministers, usually as punishment for some liberal indulgence, the shock in government is palpable.

When David Cameron was battling Eurosceptic bias in the media during the referendum campaign, he observed ruefully to an aide that he now knew what it felt like to be Labour.

Tony Blair secured a better press than any Labour leader before or since. Whether he would have governed for a decade otherwise is unknowable. That the cost was reinforcement of the parochial and reactionary media frame around matters such as immigration and Europe is certain. The control that the New Labour government was able to exert over the news agenda was formidable, and also probably the last time any such message-control system could work.

For one thing, the number of channels to influence was manageable in an analogue media environment. In the age of social media, the way information cascades from the centre of power down to the voter cannot be so easily predicted and manipulated.

But also, the Blair government's adeptness at steering the presentation of news made that very process – the dark arts of 'spin' – a story in its own right, at which point it ceased to be effective. The controversy around the case for going to war in

Iraq, the 'dodgy dossier' of evidence proving that Saddam Hussein possessed weapons of mass destruction, was so corrosive of trust in the government in part because it fitted with a growing suspicion that political reality as presented for public consumption was a tale cooked up by communications experts in league with client journalists.

The rise and fall of New Labour was a mass literacy campaign in the concepts of media manipulation. That isn't to say voters got any better at weeding out charlatans and spotting lies, only that they became more alert to the likelihood that the truth was eluding them and that anyone who appeared to communicate with managerial slickness was probably lying. One effect of that was to raise the premium on authenticity – the mode of communication that presents itself as the stylistic opposite of meticulous message control.

That allergy to conspicuously tailored messengers fed the backlash against centrism, to the benefit of figures like Farage, Corbyn and Johnson.

Audiences that were predisposed to like what populists of right and left had to say were doubly impressed because the messengers appeared to be speaking without conventional political filters. Their phrases seemed to fly straight from the gut without being checked for clearance by a communications professional somewhere in the back of the throat. That doesn't mean the phrases are any likelier to be true or that the spontaneity is even real. (In Johnson's case, the hesitations, the head-scratching and the dishevelled hair were affectations, practised to create an impression of comic improvisation.) Political authenticity means being good at appearing to do politics badly enough that people believe the person they are following is something other than a politician.

Paradoxically, the politician who basks in an aura of authenticity has a licence to be less honest than the one who performs in the old-fashioned dishonest political idiom. The charismatic showman leader's authority flows not from accurate description of reality but from compelling projection of personality. His audience will hear the ring of truth in any statement that echoes their own prejudices. He gets to deploy what Kellyanne Conway, Donald Trump's White House aide, called 'alternative facts' – fabrications that can be said to have equivalent force to actual facts if they are accepted as such by a sufficient volume of people.

Populists will always have independent media in their sights as much as they target political rivals. That is because charismatic power demands a monopoly on the decision about what is and isn't true. Journalists who deal in facts that will not bend to the gravitational field of the leader are the enemy. Under those circumstances, the conventional model of political journalism that aspires not to take sides begins to break down. To report a tyrant's words without calling him a tyrant, or to publish a liar's self-exculpation without qualifying it as a lie is non-partisan in form but complicit in practice.

It is hard for political journalism to maintain the illusion that it is acting as referee on the pitch when it is also being kicked around like a ball.

(iii) Connoisseurs of bamboozlement

Wherever there is an audience for anti-politics politicians, there will also be a warm reception for anti-media media.

Once the idea takes hold that politicians are in it for them-selves, the same suspicion extends to journalism that presents politics in any other light. Failure to denounce rottenness of the system is seen as failure to do the job properly. At its most extreme, that mistrust feeds the conspiracist fever described in Chapter 9, although a milder mistrust is prevalent.

The journalists who have the closest contact with power are despised the most because it is implicit that they know the truth and refuse to share it. The job of BBC political editor, never a relaxing gig in the past, has become an ordeal of abuse from people across the political spectrum who are convinced that the corporation is peddling propaganda against their beloved cause.

An element of moralizing censure is built into the term 'mainstream media'. It implies that any organization of sufficient scale to fund professional journalism is by definition also aligned with the political status quo and so compromised in its motives. That underestimates the importance to most journalists of breaking stories and reaching audiences. There is more integrity in the trade than its critics assume (the same is true of politics generally), but even if you presume a high level of self-serving vanity, that force will compel a reporter to expose a conspiracy sooner than collude in the cover-up.

The more insidious problem with insider journalism – and I should know, having fallen into the trap – is conflating mastery of the mechanics of how politics works behind the scenes and judgement about what politics is supposed to be achieving. Familiarity with Westminster methods can breed contempt for the opinions of amateurs. There is misplaced arrogance in thinking that politics is only *truly* understood by the people who are closest to it.

It is hard to take a detached view from an embedded position. There is a parochial kind of expertise that is valuable in a rarefied setting but not so useful beyond that. Courtiers know best what is happening at court – who is in favour with the king and who plots to unseat him – but that knowledge does not describe the condition of the kingdom.

Courtier journalism, like all reporting, has the 'story' as its tradable currency. And storytelling, in news as in fairy tales, makes a priority of character and personal conflict.

Some issues do not lend themselves to narration as plot twists in a never-ending soap opera. A fixation on personality and internecine rivalry leaves less attention for technical policy. Speculation about a Chancellor on manoeuvres, trying to undermine and eventually replace the prime minister, will excite many political journalists more than the same Chancellor's decision to adjust benefit payments that will cause material hardship to millions of people.

The soap opera is not unimportant, nor can it easily be disentangled from the policy detail. Sometimes personal vendettas between ministers are the only way to explain why a policy exists or why a U-turn has been performed to abandon it. Those things all illuminate what is going on.

But the appetite for intrigue skews the market for political news in ways that suit politicians who are adept at supplying the demand for rumour, scuttlebutt and salacious quotes, anonymously sourced. A grim but unavoidable duty I felt as a political editor was to prefer the company of MPs who dealt in personal anecdote to the ones who immersed themselves in policy.

Certain character types – the plotters and revellers in scandal

– develop better relationships with the media, and since a high media profile gets you noticed by party bosses, those relationships can be parlayed into an upward career path. Over time, that has shaped perceptions of what counts as success in politics. Dull managerial capability and command of detail are ranked lower than pugnacity and pizazz.

A system that prioritized rigour over ribaldry would never have propelled Boris Johnson all the way into Downing Street. His skills were perfectly adapted to a set-up that doesn't distinguish between the spectacle and the purpose of politics. To be successful at the show, to get the biggest ovation, is to be good at the game. And in a democracy, the winner of the game is awarded the title of people's representative. By that slippery syllogism, being good at spectacle is good politics – performance equals popularity equals democracy. It then follows that the greatest showman is also the right man for the job.

In 1988, the US journalist and writer Joan Didion observed how White House correspondents had fallen into the habit of treating the rococo artifice that had built up around the *presentation* of politics as politics itself:

American reporters 'like' covering a presidential campaign (it gets them out on the road, it has balloons, it has music, it is viewed as a big story, one that leads to the respect of one's peers, to the Sunday shows, to lecture fees and often to Washington), which is one reason why there has developed among those who do it so arresting an enthusiasm for overlooking the contradictions inherent in reporting that which occurs only in order to be reported.

To be an insider is to enjoy such fluency in the dialect of politics as salesmanship that you forget to interrogate the merit of the product. Jay Rosen, professor of journalism at New York University, has called it the 'cult of savviness'. By savviness, he means the state of being clued up, one of the cognoscenti who understands how things *really* work and so, while being phys-ically close to events, adopts a stance of sardonic distance. The savvy are never visibly distressed by a political development because that would admit having invested too much of oneself in the result. The gambler who sweats and frets is a sucker compared to the cool customer beside him who has hedged with a wager on both sides.

Rosen defined this property in a 2011 lecture:

> Prohibited from joining in political struggles, dedicated to observing what is, regardless of whether it ought to be, the savvy believe that these disciplines afford them a special view of the arena, cured of excess sentiment, useless passion, ideological certitude and other defects of vision that players in the system routinely exhibit. The savvy don't say: I have a better argument than you. They say: I am closer to reality than you. Especially if you are active in politics yourself.

The cult of savviness worships at the altar of winning elections, but is decoupled from moral questions about the ends to which victory might be put. That is not such a problem when all parties operate within a broad consensus, founded on common democratic enterprise. If it can reasonably be assumed that a government of any colour will adhere to certain basic principles of integrity and respect for dissent, there is space for journalism that cares only about who wins and makes no judgement about who *should* win.

The culture of Westminster relies heavily on the assumption that those principles exist. The cult of savviness has no vocabulary of opprobrium for a prime minister who cynically exploits other people's readiness to abide by the rules, who thinks that only the pious fuddy-duddy and the sore loser insist on scruples in a winner. That was the challenge posed by Boris Johnson, none of whose words could be fairly reported without a caveat to the effect that they might be lies.

If the only metric of success in politics is reaching the top and staying there, there is no reason to condemn a fraudster for as long as he is getting away with his fraud. A willingness to deceive is in the price, and failure is defined only by inability to sustain the deception. If someone is elected in full knowledge that he has no principles, it is hard for anyone to accuse him of failing to live up to them. The savvy observer will admire the chutzpah, deconstructing the ingenious mechanism by which cheats prosper as an innovation within the normal repertoire of politics. It makes us, in Jay Rosen's phrase, 'connoisseurs of our own bamboozlement'.

(iv) Parlour games

Boris Johnson was doubly effective as a bamboozler because the game he played was already rigged for the benefit of bluffers and chancers. He is a product of an elite education system in which the highest virtue is an ability to get on without conspicuous effort. In the public school social hierarchy, dilettantism trumps diligence and conscientious application to study is contemptible.

The ideal trajectory is a record of insouciant underperformance, punctuated with rebukes from teachers, who are then proved wrong by heroic delivery of the goods under exam conditions.

It is revealing, for example, that when Johnson wanted to disparage the legacy of David Cameron – his contemporary and rival at Eton – the term he used in cabinet* was 'girly swot'.

That attitude was (and I imagine still is) baked in at Oxford, where the tutorial system teaches above all the craft of inflating a small amount of knowledge into a makeshift edifice of argument that only needs to stay upright for the hour or so in which the student is presenting it to the tutor.

As Kuper describes it in *Chums*: 'You just had to read bits of a few books, or at least bits of a couple of books (or, if you were really pressed, one book), and then ideally lay out a bold, counterintuitive argument showing that the conventional wisdom about the topic was all wrong.' Kuper also cites Steven Hawking, who began his undergraduate studies in physics at Oxford in 1959 and observed that 'to work hard to get a better class of degree was regarded as the mark of a grey man, the worst epithet in the Oxford vocabulary'.

That attitude was still there forty years later when I was an undergraduate. It is symptomatic of an anti-intellectualism endemic in Britain's elite social strata. Partly, it expresses an aristocratic snobbery towards anyone who is obliged by lowly birth to toil – intellectualism being to the mind what hard labour is to the body. It also contains a horror of abstract ideas,

---

* The remark was contained in a leaked 2019 memo. It was much condemned on the left as an example of casual sexism. But as a window into Johnson's mind, it was doubly revealing that girlishness and studiousness were paired as twin deficiencies.

from which might spring challenges to authority and the unpicking of irrational class-based privilege.

For a certain breed of honourable member, a seat in the House of Commons is just another link in the unbroken chain of exclusive and venerable residencies that began with dispatch to boarding school in early infancy. Those people are no longer the majority in Parliament, but their sense of entitlement has reverberated there for so long that it still sets the tone.

Disregard for the virtues of academic discipline brings with it the habit of seeing politics as a competitive leisure pursuit where the prize is inscription in history books and the consolation of failure is a shorter mention in the same annals. It is what James Kirkup, a former lobby correspondent and think tank director, described in February 2022 as 'a self-regarding parlour game played by people unable or unwilling to admit that the parlour is on fire'.

The fire in question was caused by incineration of the protocols and unwritten codes of decency that uphold large parts of Britain's constitutional order. Johnson's time in Downing Street was vastly destructive in that respect (as Chapter 12 will examine). It also neutralized what had for generations been the media's most powerful weapon in holding politicians to account – the threat of shame.

Lying has been a part of the political repertoire for as long as there has been an awkward truth worth hiding. But in democratic societies with a free press and permitted opposition, bare-faced deception is also a high-stakes gamble. To be caught having made a statement orthogonal to the facts is meant to be scandalous. Careers used to be limited or ended by exposure of cynical deception. To be found to have misled Parliament is, by convention (formalized in the ministerial code of conduct), a resigning matter.

That is why spin came into existence. The art of spin is to present facts in a way that can direct or mislead an audience that is still consonant with reality. It casts a thing in a particular light, at a convenient angle. But the thing itself is not a fabrication, and the harsher light can still be applied. Spin is a game of hide-and-seek. It will describe a cut to public services as a Whitehall efficiency saving; it will bury bad news at the bottom of a press release and issue the press release late on the Friday of a bank holiday weekend. But it still makes the truth notionally available.

Spin gives the media a sporting chance to expose government in its deceptions. The innovation that Johnson brought to British politics – a lesson he learned from Trump – is that the game only works if the consequence of exposure is shame. The brazen liar can simply deny the truth altogether and, if there is an audience willing enough to indulge the fraud, stick to the lie until the media circus has moved on. There is no need to strain and make words elastic in order to depict awkward reality as you would prefer it to be when you can just snap the elastic and declare things to be as they are not.

The shameless candidate crashes through the wall of conventional disapproval and proves it is no barrier. Some of Johnson's lies did catch up with him eventually, thanks to the work of an independent press publishing awkward truths. But even then he conceded no wrong and displayed no contrition. His loyal followers assert that he was mistreated – traduced by cowards in his cabinet and hounded by malicious media. That is the view through the looking glass of a phoney revolution, where an Oxford-educated old Etonian prime minister can be cast as a victim of the Establishment; the most prolific fraudster to have occupied Downing Street can be mourned as a martyr; the truth can be turned inside out.

CHAPTER 12

THE ARSONISTS' CAKE PARTY

The inability to conceive of its own devastation will tend to be the blind spot of any culture.

Jonathan Lear

(i) Breaking glass

The Houses of Parliament are packed with poison, infested with vermin and highly combustible. That is not a metaphor. There is asbestos in the roof of the Palace of Westminster, faulty wiring behind the walls, outdated fuses, leaky pipes, rotten old wood, blocked drains and a population of impudent mice that scurry along dingy corridors, unintimidated by legislators and their staff. The building is a magnificent ruin and an accident waiting to happen. It is only licensed to operate as a workplace because fire wardens patrol on a 24-hour rota. Otherwise, health-and-safety regulations would shut it down.

Parliament has been destroyed by fire before. Twice.

In October 1834, the medieval palace that stood on the current site was levelled after underfloor heating furnaces beneath the House of Lords were left untended and raged out of control. Its replacement, the neo-Gothic behemoth that forms one of London's most famous landmarks, was badly damaged by a German bomb in 1941. The Commons chamber where MPs harangue each other today is a post-Blitz replica of the original.

The possibility of a twentieth-century upgrade was discussed and rejected. In the debate, Winston Churchill defended the old 'codes and manners' of the Commons, which he believed were inseparable from the cramped, confrontational feel of the chamber. He argued that the spirit of British democracy nested in the architecture:

> We have learned – with these so recently confirmed facts around us and before us – not to alter improvidently the physical structures which have enabled so remarkable an organism to carry on its work of banning dictatorships within this island and pursuing and beating into ruin all dictators who have molested us from outside.

Allergy to modernization has proved hard to shake. During the COVID pandemic, the government resisted the idea of MPs speaking and voting by video link, although the virus was ripping its way through the stuffy committee rooms and cramped voting lobbies. Jacob Rees-Mogg, then the minister responsible for legislative business, accepted 'hybrid' procedures reluctantly and not for long, quickly demanding that MPs 'set an example' by returning to their workplace. He bemoaned the absence of 'cut and thrust' from virtual debates.

Rees-Mogg's affection for an assertive Commons was selective. He had been less keen on Parliament the previous year, when MPs had been at loggerheads with the government over Brexit negotiations. He colluded with Boris Johnson to dissolve the legislature altogether* – an action promptly overturned as unlawful by the Supreme Court.

That episode was one among many in the Johnson era to expose a vagueness about British democracy that is its greatest vulnerability. Habits that have defined the way politics works for generations are treated as guarantees against the system being subverted. That confidence rests on Britain's self-image as a country that respects rules. Stability is supposedly baked into a constitution that has evolved by increments, in magisterial procession, not prone to fitful Gallic-style revolutions.

That notion is conveyed in Parliament as pageant – ermine robes, wigs, archaic forms of address, the State Opening, where the monarch rides to Westminster in a gilded carriage. It is mostly harmless, and more modern than it pretends to be. Much of the flummery was added in the nineteenth century, although the ceremonies recall events from 200 years earlier.

Before the official State Opening and closing of each parliamentary session,[†] there is a theatrical shutting of doors in the face of the monarch's emissary, known as Black Rod. That represents an assertion of parliamentary privilege over royal caprice, harking back to the day in 1642 when Charles I stormed into the Commons but failed to arrest MPs who were thwarting his will. Civil war and regicide followed.[‡]

---

* Long forgotten by then was the Eurosceptic claim that Brexit was necessary to restore the constitutional primacy of parliamentary sovereignty.

† The session is a block of time allocated for passing legislation, lasting for around 10–12 months, not to be mistaken for the *term*, which is the duration of the parliament itself. A parliament is dissolved for a general election, after which a new one is convened.

‡ Britain managed a decade of kinglessness before inviting Charles's son to reclaim the throne.

Those ritual re-enactments are a reminder that British democracy is old and incomplete. It is held together by loosely remembered precedent, gentleman's agreement and theatre. Those safeguards turned out to be meaningless when the government was led by a man who had mastered the ritual dances of British democracy but despised the actual rules.

Boris Johnson smuggled anarchistic contempt for historical convention into the heart of government using the perfect camouflage – the Tory party, which makes a fetish of tradition even while violating it.

Revolutionary iconoclasm used to be a predilection of the left. Ripping up the old ways, sweeping aside established institutions – those things are not conservative in the elementary sense of conserving things. There have always been Establishment revolutionaries, well heeled, supported by inherited wealth. They used to gravitate leftward, forming the cadre of 'champagne socialists' whose plans for working-class emancipation were so often frustrated by the electoral choices made by actual proletarians.

In Brexit, a champagne-quaffing set discovered they could have the frisson of Bolshevism without being made to feel like hypocrites for being rich. These Brexit Bolsheviks had their political apprenticeships in an era of prolonged and prosperous stability – Britain of the late twentieth century. Their fidgety excitement at the prospect of burning the old order down was not kept in check by any first-hand experience of the chronic disorder that history shows to be the common aftermath of revolution.

As Ivan Rogers, formerly the UK's most senior diplomat in Brussels, noted in a lecture in 2018: 'We are dealing with a political generation which has no serious experience of bad times and is, frankly, cavalier about precipitating events they cannot then control but feel they might exploit.'

These unconservative Conservatives were not ignorant of twentieth-century turmoil. On the contrary, the moral urgency of dissident toils under dictatorship was their inspiration. They resented centrist politics not for any harm it did but for the excitement it lacked. They craved the simple swashbuckling heroism of a *struggle*.

Clive James once described this restless impatience induced in some people by a surfeit of stability: 'For them, a political system which has attained a condition of vibrating stasis provides an insufficient resonance. Briefly, they find it boring. Bored, they play with fire.' James's image of recreational arson as a remedy for political boredom calls to mind George Orwell's account of left radical thought that amounts to 'playing with fire by people who don't even know that fire is hot'.

Like their Leninist counterparts on the left, Brexit Bolsheviks believed the ends justified the means – the utopian destination to be reached by way of revolution is worth any price in destruction along the way (although it is always someone else's eggs that end up broken to make the revolutionaries' omelette).

There was also synergy between the new revolutionary conservatism and old-school posh delinquency – the Bullingdon Club mentality – which takes anarchic pleasure in recreational destruction, blithely confident that any cost can be defrayed. The wrecking spirit of Brexit was a fusion of revolutionary dogma and the mannered barbarism that Evelyn Waugh, in *Decline and Fall*, characterized as 'the sound of English county families baying for broken glass'.

But wariness of violent upheaval is the ethical core of mainstream conservatism. For that reason it is meant to be suspicious of all ideology (in much the same way that it is sniffy around intellectualism). To the traditional Tory imagination, poring over blueprints for utopia is un-British; more the kind of thing you'd expect from hot-blooded continentals, whose parvenu democracies are less stable.

That isn't to say the Tories were non-ideological before Brexit. Margaret Thatcher had a doctrinal template for economic reform that her acolytes in subsequent generations turned into a sacred creed. But the pragmatic side of the Conservative tradition survived in parallel. David Cameron appealed to it in 2005 when newly elected as party leader. 'I'm not a deeply ideological person – I'm a practical person,' he said in an interview with the *Guardian*.* When asked for a definition of Cameronism, he said: 'I think that leaders in search of -isms is never a good thing.'

Eurosceptics did not wear their 'ism' – nationalism – openly. Brexit pretended to be a one-off event. Once the threshold of EU membership was crossed, the job was done. But the implied destination was a typical utopia – an idealized future where all that is disorderly and disappointing in the present is rearranged for harmony and satisfaction.

In an article for the *Sun*, Boris Johnson, Michael Gove and Labour MP Gisela Stuart jointly promised that after Brexit 'the NHS will be stronger, class sizes will be smaller, taxes lower . . . wages will be higher, fuel bills will be lower.'

---

* The fact that he was speaking to the *Guardian* at all was a mark of his intent to signal ecumenism as distinct from doctrinal purity.

Some Leaver descriptions of the world outside Brussels' jurisdiction read like the misty-eyed prognostications of the early communist visionaries. In an article for the Reaction.Life website, published two days before the 2016 referendum, Daniel Hannan, one of the most influential Conservative Eurosceptics, imagined the near future thus:

> It's 24 June, 2025, and Britain is marking its annual
> Independence Day celebration. As the fireworks stream
> through the summer sky, still not quite dark, we wonder why
> it took us so long to leave. The years that followed the 2016
> referendum didn't just reinvigorate our economy, our
> democracy and our liberty. They improved relations with our
> neighbours.

He went on to forecast that the UK would 'lead the world in biotech, law, education, the audio-visual sector, financial services and software'. It would be a centre for the production of driverless cars, but its older industries would also be enjoying a renaissance: steel, cement, paper, plastics, ceramics.*

The failure of Brexit to fulfil those promises will never be acknowledged by the architects of the revolution. This, too, is consistent with the Bolshevik mentality, which has a limitless capacity for generating excuses. The plan itself is never wrong, just implemented badly or blocked by saboteurs. It is the balm of self-deception that Western socialists applied to their wounded egos when the communist regimes they had vaunted

---

* As I write, it is not yet 2025, so Hannan's vision still has time. But it is worth noting that he published almost exactly the same article in the *Daily Telegraph* a year earlier, and in that version paradise was obtained by 2020.

as havens of proletarian welfare ossified into dictatorship and crumbled into bankruptcy.

In some Tories, the Bolshevik temperament was on display before Brexit. David Cameron once described Michael Gove as 'a bit of a Maoist – he believes that the world makes progress through the process of creative destruction'.* Gove kept a portrait of Lenin in his ministerial office. He attributed the choice to 'an element of humour and irony . . . as well as a reminder of the importance of making a difference'.†

The revolutionary strain of conservatism was on a collision course with traditionalism. Gove and Cameron ended up on opposing sides. Remain-supporting MPs and the Menshevik tendency that preferred milder terms of departure from the EU were purged.

The Brexit utopians, being a cult of rage against the status quo, were ill-equipped for success. Getting what they wanted was psychologically disorienting. They reached their Promised Land too quickly. The technical fact of legal separation from the EU was done by the end of January 2020. Once Johnson's deal with Brussels was signed, there wasn't much further out of Europe Britain could practically get.

There was Northern Ireland still to haggle over. For Euro-sceptic fanatics, the compromise that bound Ulster to EU regulations for the sake of avoiding a new land border with the

---

* 'Creative destruction' is an allusion to the Austrian-born political economist Joseph Schumpeter, whose theories of capitalist evolution developed into one of the most influential critiques of Marxism in the twentieth century.

† The appeal to irony as an excuse for displaying an icon of murderous dictatorship resembles the moral slipperiness of alt-right trolls who strike fascist poses and call it edgy. It is doubtful Gove would have been so glib about right-wing tyrants, or hung their portraits on his wall.

Republic of Ireland was an affront; a portion of sovereignty pinched from Britannia's pocket as she fled Brussels. But for most English Leave voters, that was an arcane dispute.

The revolution had to shift gears quickly from promises to excuses. The pandemic provided a period of cover, disrupting supply chains and stalling trade. Russia's war against Ukraine was also a feasible explanation for economic woes that swerved reference to Britain's self-exclusion from continental markets. But the conspicuous absence of material reward from the great liberation was harder to explain.

In June 2022, to celebrate Queen Elizabeth II's Platinum Jubilee, Johnson announced a restored right for shopkeepers to display produce exclusively in imperial weights and measures (a requirement for metric labelling being an old Eurosceptic grievance). Even his fans could hear the difference between a drum being beaten and a barrel being scraped.

In revolution, as in everything else, Johnson was only ever a dilettante. His personal mission had been to reach Downing Street. He was not temperamentally cut out for long struggles. For him, Brexit was an essay-crisis utopia, cobbled together from skim-read history and bluffer's guide economics, submitted for marking by an indulgent press, which awarded him top marks in national salvation.

Brussels directives had not caused the social and economic distress that was exploited so effectively to win the referendum, so the promised dividend in sovereignty was not convertible into improved conditions for Leave voters. The areas that had most craved change were among those worst affected by the cost-of-living crisis that Brexit did nothing to alleviate and much to exacerbate. Disruption to trade and constraints on labour markets fed inflation, visiting disproportionate pain on some of the least resilient places. Brexit was poison sold as antidote.

A revolution that has achieved its defining purpose while meeting none of its higher goals condemns its leaders to a cycle of endless grievance-mining. They must be always drilling deeper into culture wars and nationalist vendettas in search of new reserves of energy to fuel their project. They are condemned to be arsonists masquerading as firefighters, stirring social division and pretending their purpose is national unity.

(ii) Cakeism

In the beginning, Brexit was a word full of contradictions. Boris Johnson was the word made flesh. His ebullient optimism was ideal for propagandizing a utopian vision, while his bumbling toff shtick deodorized the whiff of chaos. He made a jape of upheaval, as if rupture with Britain's allies and nearest trading partners were no less an adventure and no more a hazard than a Bertie Wooster escapade. He was Brexit's biggest lie incarnate – that you could break everything and also keep everything the same.

Before the referendum campaign, Johnson's theatrical talent had been dedicated to the only cause he could care about for any sustained period – himself. It needed people like Gove and Dominic Cummings, the former Vote Leave strategist brought into Downing Street in 2019, to provide the rigid ideological mould into which the wobbly jelly of Johnson's gut politics could be poured.

They made a potent team. Without Johnson's loose charm,

the swivel-eyed ideologues would have struggled to sell their revolution to the masses. Without the Bolshevik steel, Johnson would not have had the discipline to turn his ravenous appetite for power into a plan for getting it.

Before he had a plan, he had his kitschy, end-of-pier Churchill tribute act. To the extent that he had a belief system, it consisted in faith that intractable problems are solved when great men appoint themselves as the solution. His response to technical objections was to dismiss them as symptoms of deficient optimism and flaccid will.

'My policy on cake is pro having it and pro eating it,' he would say, subverting the famous proverb. It was a favourite catchphrase before Brexit.* He even tried it out as a defence of Britain's EU membership in a draft article, never published, endorsing the Remain side in the 2016 referendum. But the line really took off as a device for dismissing doubt about the credibility of Britain's negotiating aims in Brussels. The plan was riddled with impossible combinations: Britain would not suffer from Brexit because it would retain the benefits of EU membership, and also because EU membership conferred no benefits worth preserving. Britain could leave a trading bloc without loss of trade. It could have different customs regimes for Great Britain and Northern Ireland without a pesky customs border between them. The doctrine that made it all seem possible was cakeism.

'I want you to see this as a cakeist treaty,' Johnson said of the post-Brexit trade deal he signed in December 2020.

---

* Johnson recycles his favourite lines in different contexts. The twist on a proverbial prohibition on having cake and eating it has been attributed to him in interviews and profiles dating back at least to 2008.

Cakeism was more than a formula for wishing away diplomatic and economic complexity on the European front. It sprawled. It described Johnson's inability to sustain a strategy for handling the coronavirus pandemic, or indeed any governing challenge. He wanted to limit COVID infections without imposing draconian restraints on individual freedoms. He wanted a programme for 'levelling up' – transferring resources to his recently captured electoral properties in former Labour heartlands – without having to tax his Home Counties Tory heartlands; he wanted a 'green industrial revolution' that presupposed massive increases in public investment, but without offending Tory ambitions for a smaller state.

To serve in Johnson's cabinet, ministers were expected to be cakeists. They had to embody the paradox of a conservative revolution – the contradiction inherent in harnessing anti-Establishment insurrection to keep the old ruling party in power.

As electoral strategy, cakeism was the heir to turn-of-the-century centrism in that it built a coalition of voters across conventional left–right divides. It allowed the Tories to be the party of 'red wall' towns and the true-blue shires.* But cakeism is unlike most political doctrines in its knowing insistence on the impossible. It is a pastiche ideology that mocks the conventional requirement for coherence and consistency.

That was politically feasible with Brexit because most people's experience of what the EU did and how it worked was vague. The lie that it would be all upside was durable because

---

* To what extent Johnson's victory was a seismic realignment of cultural allegiance or a spasmodic reaction to the combination of Brexit impasse and Corbyn as the other option for prime minister is something that future elections will reveal.

the downside had a slow burn and was then camouflaged by the pandemic.

When confronted with a deadly virus, cakeism was a disaster. The effect of the disease could not be deferred or belittled with boosterism. None of the tools of Westminster craft that had served Johnson and his generation in their previous careers was of practical use against a microscopic pathogen. It could not be campaigned against, slandered by anonymous briefing, outlawed, bullied or bribed. The virus didn't care about its reputation or its appeal to the electorate. It didn't care if you lied about it.

An auxiliary problem was Johnson's rakish libertine streak – licentious appetite dressed as respectable philosophy of freedom. It didn't amount to anything so rigid as an ideology, more a buttery layer in the cake. He extrapolated a generalized view of the British psyche from his own aversion to following rules. He styled himself as the champion of Merrie England, scourge of regulatory fusspots, who could vaporize gloom with the radiant heat of his optimism. That made it hard to adjust to the role of killjoy-in-chief, shuttering pubs and cancelling Christmas.

Being a coward under fire, the prime minister sought human shields. He found scientists. In televised press conferences, he ostentatiously deferred to his chief advisers on matters medical and statistical. Eagerness to evade any blame for unpleasantness was etched on his face.

The repeated claim that the government was being 'led by the science' during the pandemic was half true. Johnson took his scientific instruction, but in the manner of a recalcitrant child pushing vegetables around a plate.

Had it not been for the swift development of vaccines and their competent delivery, his time in office might have been even shorter. It is telling that the peak of his opinion-poll ratings followed his hospitalization with COVID. He was valued more as a mascot, an emblem of the peril everyone felt at that moment, than as a leader who might get stuff done. He rose to the top by getting people to like him. It was all downhill once they got to know him.

The trait people come to dislike in a leader is usually the origin of their previous appeal inverted. The stolidity that once recommended Theresa May and Gordon Brown turned robotic. The charm of Tony Blair and David Cameron went from smooth to slippery. With Johnson, it was the celebration of unruliness, the maverick disregard for convention. His cavalier spirit was welcome when the job was breaking through the Brexit impasse. It soured into arrogance, dereliction of duty, pathological estrangement from the truth and, in the case of Downing Street parties during lockdown, law-breaking.

At his most effective, Johnson enacted a cartoonish caricature of himself that allowed the roguish incompetence to hide in plain sight. Amateurishness and inattention to detail were components of the authenticity that meant, paradoxically, he could be a populist with no obligation to sound like the people.

He transcended his elite status by camping it up as 'Boris'. That character activated something in the English psyche that derives reassurance from an old-fashioned styling of power, while stripping it of the hauteur that can alienate people from posh authority.

But the accompanying temperament was unsuited to decision-making in government. Johnson liked to be liked and hated direct confrontation. He had no qualms about betraying people behind their backs, but a horror of upsetting them to their faces. MPs would come out of meetings in Downing Street happy because their leader had acquiesced to some demand, unaware that he had made an opposite promise to their rivals in a meeting earlier the same day. He dealt with problems by letting them run out of control. He handled dilemmas by neglecting them until the choice became perversely easier because there were fewer options left. If he waited long enough, there might be only one. That was the method that produced a Brexit deal with Brussels (albeit a bodged one that did not take long to unravel), and it was the technique that was applied to life-or-death decisions over pandemic restrictions.

In testimony to a parliamentary committee in 2021, Cummings described a conversation in which Johnson admitted that disorder was his preferred modus operandi. 'Chaos isn't that bad,' the prime minister was reported as saying. 'Chaos means that everyone has to look to me to see who's in charge.'* That was the vanity of an authoritarian personality cult, stripped of any dictatorial purpose beyond the fact of being in charge. (Johnson had said as a child that his ambition was to become 'world king'.)

There is an arrogance common to aristocratic and revolutionary elites that view themselves as authors of history

---

* In another version of that conversation, Cummings has Johnson say, 'I'm quite happy to live with the chaos because then everyone will stick to the king – which is me.' The different renderings might cast doubt on Cummings' memory or reliability as a witness, but the underlying managerial dynamic is confirmed privately by many people who have worked for and alongside Johnson.

rather than mere characters within it. They claim to be acting beneficently on behalf of the common people, but that paternalism contains a moral detachment that decays into contempt. That was the origin of the 'Partygate' scandal. It sprang from a presumption that Great Helmsmen are not bound by the rules they make for little people.

That attitude was an ingredient in Johnson's charm when it was expressed as defiance of Brussels or pettifogging parliamentarians. But in the context of pandemic restrictions, the people made to look like fools were the ones who had obeyed the rules, often at personal cost, missing weddings, funerals, physical contact with grandchildren and dying relatives.

Johnson's downfall was baked into cakeism. Its combination of nationalism, Bolshevism and old-school Toryism with a sprinkle of charisma on top was a recipe for failure. It defined itself by a deception that is intrinsic to all such ideological projects – the claim that hard choices can be avoided. One day, the cake has to be shared, rationed, and people notice who gets the largest portion.

The candidate who triumphed by treating everything as a joke was caught laughing at his voters. The light changed; the impish grin darkened into a sneer; the populist lost his people; the polarities of his magnetism flipped; and the force that was once attraction turned repulsive.

(iii) Good chaps

Corruption takes hold in all revolutionary regimes when they lose ideological momentum. It is the decadent stage once a party elite have understood that utopia is unattainable but are enjoying the trappings of power too much to break the bad news to the people in whose name they seized it.

There is a squeamishness in Britain about calling corruption by its name. The preferred term is 'sleaze' – a catch-all word whose effect is thinned by being spread too wide. It covers every shade of venality from sexual indiscretion to misallocation of funds, via grey areas of lobbying and the casual trade in commercial favours for political cronies. That last proclivity has its own anaesthetic neologism – 'chumocracy'. Chumminess sounds milder, less jagged than crookedness.

Johnson's regime explored every byway of sleaze. The offence that finally provoked Conservative MPs to unseat him was his tolerance of alleged sexual harassment by a party whip (and his subsequent lying about it). But before that, there had been the parties – and the lying about them – leading to the indignity of Johnson becoming the first sitting prime minister to receive a criminal sanction from the police.*

What else? He tried to scrap the independent office of the parliamentary standards commissioner after its investigation found a Conservative MP guilty of breaching rules on 'paid advocacy' (abusing the office to lobby for private clients). He lost two advisers on ethics in disputes over the ministerial code – a manual for government propriety that turns out to be worthless if neither its spirit nor its letter are honoured in Downing Street. Johnson amended the code, excising the expectation that ministers who fall foul of it should resign. His updated version dispensed with a preamble that had

---

* Others might have broken the law before him but were not caught or charged.

required 'honesty, integrity, transparency and accountability' in government.

There is an obvious flaw in a system for policing good behaviour in a prime minister when that prime minister is also the author and arbiter of the rules. But the letter of the code was never meant to be the final word on government conduct. Historically, the boundaries of propriety were intuitive, moderated by conscience, honour and good sportsmanship. These virtues were theoretically instilled by the aristocratic ethos of *noblesse oblige* and cultivated by the public school system. It was an apparatus summarized by the historian and peer Peter Hennessy as 'the good chap' theory of government.

Good chaps would know the limits of decency, and as long as Whitehall and Downing Street were populated with the right kind of person, beastliness and barbarism could never prosper. In 1879, William Gladstone described the British constitution in similar terms, asserting that it 'presumes more boldly than any other the good sense and good faith of those who work in it'.

Johnson might as well have been genetically engineered as a stress test for that proposition. He was bred to bypass informal checks and balances. He had the exemplary external presentation of a good chap – white and male; Eton and Oxford – but none of the interior restraints that those ethnographic criteria were supposed to advertise. The 'Boris' persona was a camouflage of repute, perfect for a pattern of fraud that would never have been tolerated for so long by so many if it hadn't been perpetrated in the accent of England's ruling class.

British financial corruption is modest by global standards.

Public administration is not routinely lubricated by back-handers. Officials do not take jobs just for the pilfering opportunities. If you are arrested, the police will not automatically take a bribe to release you. In January 2023, the UK ranked 18th in the annual global chart of perceived corruption compiled by Transparency International. (A high placement indicates honesty and the bottom of the table is reserved for failed states and war zones.)

Johnson's regime was not rotten on the scale of khaki-clad tyrants who siphon millions into Swiss bank accounts, build themselves marble palaces and relieve themselves in gold toilets. In the genre of opulent self-indulgence, there was only a grubby business around lavish wallpaper for the private quarters in Downing Street, financed by a Tory donor. There was also an unrealized plan to install a £150,000 tree house at Chequers for use by the prime minister's infant son.

It is a measure of how complacent British politics is about corruption that during the pandemic, the government set up an official 'VIP channel' for public procurement of medical materials. The result was a bonanza of cowboy deals and cavalier contracts awarded to contacts of senior Conservatives.* A lot of the equipment thus acquired – worth £2.8 billion; around a fifth of the total spend – was later found to be unfit for use in the NHS. In January 2022, the High Court ruled that circumventing the normal procedures with the VIP lane had been illegal. But the offence hardly registered in the clamour of competing scandal around Downing Street at the time.

---

* At least £1.6 billion of contracts was awarded on the basis of contacts provided by just 10 Conservative MPs.

A decorative crust of Westminster habit covers the gap between practices banned by law and normalized informal dodginess. Every now and then, a scandal breaks the seal, as it did in the case of parliamentary expenses. Before the receipts were leaked, the routine of casually topping up MPs' salaries had been so established that no one seemed to think it constituted an abuse. Few of the transactions were fraudulent in a strictly legal sense.

The whole business of peerages – party leaders sending their donors and pals to the upper chamber of Parliament – is a grotesque monument to complacency. To invent such a system and call it democracy would be absurd, but once installed, it seems impossible to dismantle – a scam badged as tradition and protected by ritual. (The explicit sale of honours was made illegal in 1925, but appointments to the House of Lords are still transactional.)

Cronyism is not the exclusive vice of Conservatives. Labour politicians are quite capable of abusing power when and wherever they monopolize it long enough to have the opportunity. But the Tories have a more settled relationship with government, and a more instinctive sense of entitlement to be there. Britain had a Conservative prime minister for two in every three years of the twentieth century. Labour got a 10-year head start in the twenty-first century and already the Tories have governed longer.

That formidable record of winning elections, combined with a winner-takes-all constitution, breeds an arrogance that goes fist in glove with the hereditary belief in aristocratic entitlement to rule. A British prime minister in command of a parliamentary majority enjoys a suite of powers that is the envy of presidents in modern republics, where executive fiat is checked by the separation of powers and senates are elected.*

The House of Lords often checks the will of Downing Street, but with the diminished heft of an appointed chamber. For the Commons to reject government legislation, it usually takes a rebellion among MPs of the ruling party. Since the ruling party is more often than not the Tories, the central conflict in British politics is frequently a grudge match between factions of conservatism.

Four times since the Brexit referendum a new prime minister has been installed by the Tory party without the rest of the country being consulted. Theresa May and Rishi Sunak were appointed by a caucus of MPs. Boris Johnson and Liz Truss were empowered by ballots of Conservative members, accounting for no more than 0.5 per cent of eligible nationwide voters.

Britain's democratic culture is strong enough that prime ministers chosen by that method soon feel bereft of a proper mandate (and the opposition will nag them about it). But the habit of sloughing the robes of high office from one set of Tory shoulders to another reinforces a sense that the party's relationship with government is more natural than the one Labour might form from time to time; that the political system and conservatism have evolved in symbiosis.

There is a tacit assumption that the stability of British

---

* The way Britain's constitution presents very few institutional checks on executive power has been described as 'elective dictatorship'. The phrase is often attributed to the former Tory minister Quintin Hogg (aka Lord Hailsham), via a lecture he delivered in 1976, but in fact it is many decades older.

democracy, residing in its oldest institutions, is a property of Conservative rule. Toryism is so ingrained in Establishment politics as to be practically a muscle memory by which power is exercised. The corrupting effect is similar to the one that took hold in authoritarian communist states, where the ruling party elite awarded itself the exclusive authority to decide what was doctrinally correct and what was heretical. In a one-party state, right and wrong are defined as whatever the politburo says they are, and they tend to judge their own actions generously.

But Britain is not a one-party state. There have been times when England has felt like one (Scotland too, but under a different party). Then there are times when arrogance bursts the banks of dignity and the contents of a political sewer are washed out into the open by the hubristic flood. It happened in the mid nineties, when John Major's government was overrun by a tide of 'sleaze'.

When Conservative ministers dole out contracts and fiscal favours for their friends, they do not think of themselves as corrupt. They are insulated from that perception by a feeling of natural alignment with the constitutional order – the innate feeling of *belonging* in power. The old networks of patronage and privilege are woven so tightly into the Westminster upholstery that decay can pass as decor.

When Johnson was challenged at a press conference in November 2021 over his handling of a lobbying scandal, he declared that Britain was 'not remotely a corrupt country', and it is likely he believed it, because his idea of a 'corrupt country' is somewhere foreign, a banana republic, some sharp-elbowed, queue-barging nation, less blessed than Britain is with gentleman administrators and all-round good sports.*

The last rites on the 'good chaps' theory were read on Tuesday, 12 April 2022 by Lord Hennessy himself. It was the day that Johnson received his fine from the police and read a carefully scripted, precisely disingenuous apology for TV cameras, minimizing his offence.

Hennessy noted the moment in his diary as one that 'will be forever remembered as a dark bleak day for public and political life'. He described Johnson as 'the great debaser in modern times of decency ... and of our constitutional conventions'. In breaking the law and misleading Parliament about it, Johnson, the 'wrong 'un in chief', had sullied his office like no other prime minister, 'turning it into an adventure playground for one man's narcissistic vanity'.

Johnson was never shamed into resignation or brought down by the opposition. He was defenestrated by his own MPs, not because they were morally affronted by their reprobate leader's behaviour, but because they looked at opinion polls and by-election results and concluded that he had become an electoral liability. Trampling principles of democracy was clumsy, but to threaten the Tory hold on power was a capital crime.

---

* This is the same parochial complacency, encountered in Part One, that encourages Conservatives to indulge every mythological cliché from the nationalist canon while believing that nationalism is an affliction of insecure, arriviste political cultures.

(iv) The emperor's old clothes

No sooner had the Conservatives rid themselves of Johnson than many of them started to feel remorse. This was not because he had managerial skills they missed in Downing Street, but because so much of the party's self-esteem and reputation was invested in the pretence that he had governed well. (A hapless successor made that illusion easier to sustain.)

Admitting the extent to which Johnson had abused his office would have meant owning the mistake of putting him there in the first place. Besides, it was hard to denounce him as a serial fraudster without conceding, at least by implication, that Brexit was his greatest fraud. It was more comforting to think that his critics had got needlessly carried away; that he had been stabbed in the back and traduced by bloodthirsty media. But a more universal psychological mechanism was also at work. When chill winds of reality threatened to expose Tory delusion they sought insulation in more layers of denial.

The story of the emperor's new clothes is commonly told as a parable of stupid vanity pricked by innocent candour. The narcissist ruler is persuaded by a pair of crooks posing as tailors that a magnificent robe has been woven for him from magic cloth. Only good and wise men can see it. Afraid to admit that he sees nothing, the despot pretends to admire the suit and wears it on a parade. No one dares say the obvious thing – that the monarch is stark naked – because all fear exposure as wicked fools who can't see the enchanted fabric. Then a child speaks up. The emperor has no clothes! Everyone suddenly grasps this self-evident truth and the whole town takes up the child's cry.

But that isn't the end. Hans Christian Andersen's original fable concludes with a lesson in the persistence of delusion in the face of ridicule: 'The emperor shivered, for he suspected they were right. But he thought, "This procession has got to go on." So he walked more proudly than ever, as his noblemen held high the train that wasn't there at all.'

Pride is not the only reason why naked emperors and their flatterers carry on marching. Stupidity, greed and fear play their part. Mediocrities who have risen further than their capabilities should allow, having made their careers writing rave reviews of magic fabric, dread losing their jobs if the truth is acknowledged. When the whole court has been turned over to the production and sale of bogus finery, regime change carries the threat of repercussions – demands for a refund; pursuit of redress through the courts.

Johnson was a naked emperor and Brexit was his procession. The show stayed on the road because Britain has a political system where democracy, imperious pageant and Conservative entitlement to rule come as a bundle.

Under those unique conditions, he could be removed from office, ostensibly because the government was failing, and replaced with a prime minister who had served him loyally in that same government and refused to repudiate her former patron. The installation of Liz Truss in Downing Street was another turn of the phoney revolutionary cycle – continuity dressed up as change; more revving of rhetorical engines while the wheels spun frictionlessly and the country sank deeper into a political and economic quagmire.

It was a ridiculous spectacle and a parody of democratic accountability, but also consistent with the normal operation of a democracy that has theatrical absurdity in its DNA, scribbling its rules on goatskin parchment and keeping its constitutional checks and balances in a dressing-up box alongside crowns, rods and baubles.

Britain likes to think of itself as the world's cradle of civilized government and the Palace of Westminster as 'the mother of parliaments'. The resilience of a democracy is apparently measured by its vintage. Maturity is strength. That is sometimes true, but age can also bring rot. The supporting timbers can look splendid without being sturdy.

Brexit was not a full-frontal assault on that structure. It imported the ethos of a revolutionary junta to squat in the shell of a democratic constitution that was itself whittled out of decrepit monarchy. State power was notionally still operated by the traditional levers, according to familiar practice. But permission to take charge of those levers was reserved for those who met the requisite standard of doctrinal purity, as judged by the revolutionary Blue Guards.

Liz Truss became prime minister because she understood how to game that dynamic. She had campaigned for Remain in 2016, but recanted quickly and cultivated instead alliance with the European Research Group – the commissariat of Brexit belief in the parliamentary Tory party.

Rishi Sunak, Truss's rival in the 2022 contest, had been a Brexit supporter from the start, and yet perversely found himself cast as the more Remain-ish of the candidates. Brexit by then had crossed from being a project of statecraft to a state of mind. Sunak's slick managerial style and calls for fiscal sobriety aligned him with the pre-revolutionary Tory tradition. His wealth, marriage to the daughter of an Indian tech billionaire and demeanour of a man at ease with business-class travel had a touch of globalism;* of what Theresa May had meant by a 'citizen of nowhere'. His resignation from Johnson's cabinet had been instrumental in the prime minister's downfall, and since 'Boris' and Brexit were extensions of the same brand, betraying the man amounted in Conservative eyes to disparaging the mission.

By contrast, Truss ran as a dyed-in-the-wool Brexit Bolshevik, a Johnsonian and a cakeist. She refused to engage with the painful choices that would shortly be facing her government. She denounced the economic record of the administration in which she had made her own career. She promised to jettison the 'failed orthodoxies' that had plagued Britain, as if some other party had been responsible for the blight. But she spared Johnson's personal degeneracy in her repudiation of everything that came before her. His legacy (the one she was also pledging to discard) would be safe in her hands.

Also in conformity with the historical pattern of revolution, the Trussite iteration preferred brute force to popular persuasion. The new prime minister imagined she could use her hand-me-down mandate to pursue an agenda woven from the most fanatical strands of right-wing economic doctrine. This was the opportunity afforded by a Brexit model that would never have won a referendum campaign had it been declared as the explicit purpose of the project.

Since escape from Europe had been achieved, the utopian

---

* There isn't compelling evidence that racism was the reason why Sunak failed to become prime minister on the first attempt, but if it featured in that contest against Truss, it was here – sublimated into the more subtle prejudice against cosmopolitanism.

cartographers had to draw up a new destination – the land of economic growth reached by way of tax cuts and deregulation. Here was the same Bolshevik spirit, but Brexit was now the means. The end was pushed back over the horizon.

The enemy was unchanged. Writing in the *Daily Telegraph*, David Frost, Boris Johnson's former Brexit negotiator, defended Truss's plans as a courageous march into battle with 'the economic establishment', in whose ranks he placed the International Monetary Fund (which had recently fretted over the government's incontinent budget), the European Commission, former prime ministers and Bank of England governors, the *Financial Times*, *The Economist* and 'the whole ghastly crew that thinks the West inevitably faces stagnation and decline'.

With phrases that would not have been out of place in a Leninist pamphlet from a hundred years earlier, Frost denounced the fetishists of 'stability'. Political and economic equilibrium were not desirable (regardless of what the public wanted) because they amounted to 'the quiet stability of the grave'.* What was needed, Frost fulminated from his plush sinecure in the House of Lords, was the 'constant churn and change that comes with dynamic capitalism'.

In the only keynote speech Truss made to a Conservative conference as prime minister, she widened the attack even further. She planned to jolt the economy into surges of productivity. Anyone who quailed at her disruptive methods belonged to an 'anti-growth coalition', comprising opposition parties, trade unions, think tanks, 'talking heads', environmental

---

* Here there is an echo of the 'vibrating stasis' that Clive James identified as the cause of boredom that provokes ideological arson.

activists and people who 'taxi from north London townhouses to the BBC studio to dismiss anyone challenging the status quo'. (Such geographic precision was necessary to avoid accidentally locating Truss's fine *south* London townhouse in the insidious network of counter-revolutionary subterfuge.)

Johnson had wanted to cajole the nation to sunlit uplands. Truss preferred the forced march – the method of populism without the ballast of popularity. Both techniques were doomed.

Utopia must always stay beyond view, a figment of the ideologues' imagination somewhere over yonder. The route can change, the journey time can be revised, but the one thing that must never be admitted, the humiliating truth, is that the compass is broken, the map useless and the leader lost.

When Truss's government imploded, Tory MPs sent for Sunak, the rival she had beaten only months before, bypassing a consultation of party members to ensure a quick succession and avert a Johnsonist revanche. That manoeuvre contained some recognition of deficient splendour in the imperial wardrobe, but not much.

The new prime minister's mandate was all the more threadbare and his prospectus unoriginal. He preached fiscal discipline to fill the budget hole excavated by Truss's explosive ideological experiments while giving permission for culture warrior parades along the old Brexit marching route to satisfy his party's restive nationalists. The cut of Sunak's cloth was more sober than anything styled by his predecessor but it was still cut to a design of magical thinking.

And thus the invisible fabric passes from one Emperor to the next. The procession must continue. The revolution is never complete. It has just been delayed. The plan was never wrong, only implemented improperly. The wondrous material will be shown to better effect with a new leader whose stride will be more prudent yet also more purposeful. It just needs a new model to display those brilliant properties that quislings and saboteurs refuse to admire. One more stride along Downing Street to silence the rising chorus of scorn and derision from people who say there is nothing there.

Part Four

PERSPECTIVES

CHAPTER 13

THE REVENGE OF HISTORY

With too much confidence and too little reflection we put the twentieth century behind us and strode boldly into its successor swaddled in self-serving half-truths: the triumph of the West, the end of History, the unipolar American moment, the ineluctable march of globalization and the free market.

Tony Judt

(i) A mundane miracle

When Britain went to war with Germany in 1939, Clive Campbell was 16 years old; too young to fight. When he came of age for conscription two years later, he enlisted in his home town of Derby, but was never sent into combat. He had trained as an electrical engineer, which counted as one of the 'reserved occupations' – trades that were needed on the home front. Only after the Nazis had surrendered was Clive deployed to Germany, keeping the lights on and repairing the electrics for the occupying Allied forces. He was stationed in Itzehoe, a small town north-west of Hamburg.

There, Clive's eye was caught by Ilse Buch, a pretty 19-year-old German girl who spoke passable English. She worked in a hotel, which must have catered exclusively for military personnel. There wasn't any tourism in post-war Itzehoe. It was the site of a camp for 'displaced persons' – holding pens that were set up across occupied Germany, Italy and Austria to process the millions of refugees, mostly Eastern Europeans, who had fled the fighting or been liberated from concentration camps.

Ilse was a Berliner originally, but had spent the war as an evacuee, in rural safekeeping in the Sudetenland – the strip of Czechoslovakia annexed by the Third Reich in 1938. German children and youths were hosted in hotels and schools. They had lessons and leisure activities – sport, music, games – all under the guidance of a team leader from the Hitler Youth. Only those of authenticated 'German blood' were allowed.

Older boys received paramilitary training. Girls like Ilse were put to work on the land. She once injured a finger picking potatoes and fretted about falling behind in her chores, but had no complaints otherwise. She did not resent the austere lifestyle. She was discovering the thrill of being a teenager away from home at what sounded – the way she later told it – like a jolly Girl Guide camp. But run by Nazis.

There aren't many details about Clive and Ilse's courtship. They both loved classical music and attended the same concerts in Itzehoe, first separately, then together, and soon inseparably. They married in 1947 and moved in with Clive's mother in Derby. The older Mrs Campbell was not thrilled by this development. She had lined up a respectable English girl to be her daughter-in-law, and her plans had been foiled by the blonde usurper, imported from enemy territory. But Ilse was strong-willed and not going anywhere. A chilly truce was reached.

Half a century passed. The couple moved south, first to Crawley, then on to Brighton. Ilse taught at primary schools, eventually becoming a head teacher. She adopted the name Margaret, to sound more English, although friends and family knew her as Liz. Clive passed on his electrician's trade teaching at technical colleges. When I met the couple, they had retired to a manicured suburban cul-de-sac in Haywards Heath, a West Sussex market town. They had grandchildren, one of whom married me.

The Third Reich came up rarely in conversation with my wife's grandmother. I remember only one occasion, when she said that after the war, her family had been appalled to learn about atrocities committed by their countrymen in honour of the flag they had saluted. I never pressed the point. Liz, formerly Ilse, had welcomed me enthusiastically into her family and was a loving, generous great-grandmother to my children. It was somehow never the right moment to interrogate her adolescence under a regime that would have made the existence of those children a crime. She died in 2011.

Clive, my children's great-grandfather, also didn't talk much about the war or its aftermath. He never mentioned the refugee processing station at Itzehoe. I later learned that it had mostly housed people from the Baltic region. Some had been freed from Nazi camps and some had fled the fighting. Maybe a distant cousin of mine from Linkuva passed through the town while Ilse and Clive were courting. Or maybe somewhere in that refugee camp was the distant cousin's murderer, a nationalist partisan, escaping the westward march of the Red Army.

Coincidences like that are the stuff of novels and movies. My story is constrained by a scarcity of known facts. I do know that my two daughters spent their infancy in a Europe where the absence of war felt completely normal, although it was exceptional in the long view of history. I know also that their family tree, just two generations up, has one branch that feared Nazis and another that followed them; that it took cumulative migrations across thousands of miles for those branches to intertwine, and also a continental reconciliation that feels all the more miraculous because it became mundane.

Europe has tens of millions of such children, the fruit of peaceful integration. They did not have a vote, or a voice, when Britain opted to quit the union of nations that was founded to curate that conciliatory principle. But I voted with them in mind and so, I am sure, did Clive. He was against Brexit; he found the whole concept appalling. By 2016, he was growing frail and needed the help of a walking frame to get to a polling station to cast his ballot for Remain. He died in 2017, a proud citizen of a place called Europe.

(ii) Post-post-war

There are many different ways of defining the era that started with the defeat of the Axis powers in 1945. Historians disagree as to whether it amounts to a single period or a succession of phases.* But one term captures the whole – 'post-war'.

No one seeing that term needs to ask which war. The 'post'

---

* In economic policy, there is a distinct crunching of gears in the seventies, when a Keynesian consensus unravelled, and a decisive shift at the end of the Cold War. We're coming to that shortly.

prefix doesn't mean conflict in Europe was abolished. There was plenty of violence in the second half of the twentieth century but no repetition of the mechanized carnage that defined the first half. That difference, and the determination to maintain it by means of diplomacy, international law and organizations for the mediation of disputes between nations, is what post-war means.

It refers to a set of assumptions about the way the world works, and to the institutions and habits of liberal democracy in rich and powerful countries that are meant to keep things working that way.

A loose synonym is 'Western', although that has a different inflection. Post-war refers to a world that remembers the horrors of fascism enough to make sure they stay buried in the past. The West has an implied antagonist in the East. It derives its meaning from the ideological confrontation that shaped international affairs for more than four decades after 1945. The Cold War effected an alignment of post-war values and geography. The bedrock belief of this *political* West was that democracy, resting on a cushion of capitalist prosperity, was the most effective system ever created for arranging happy, peaceful societies, and by extension, morally superior to any alternative.

That confidence was puffed into geostrategic cockiness when the Berlin Wall fell in 1989. The elimination of communist regimes from the race for global supremacy left the Western model unchallenged and, in the eyes of its champions, insuperable. It was the point of benign social, economic and political equilibrium to which human civilization inevitably tended.

That idea is commonly, and sometimes unfairly, summarized as the 'end of history' thesis, as set out in a book* by the political scientist Francis Fukuyama in 1992. Fukuyama did not claim that the wheels of history had stopped turning, nor did he assert that liberal democracy and market capitalism were immortal. He observed the absence of credible alternatives, since every effort to make Marxism work as a practical recipe for government had led to penury and tyranny:

> What we are witnessing is not just the end of the Cold War,
> or a passing of a particular period of post-war history, but
> the end of history as such: that is, the end point of mankind's
> ideological evolution and the universalization of Western
> liberal democracy as the final form of human government.

The two decades following the fall of the Iron Curtain did fulfil a lot of the advertised benefits of capitalism and democracy for millions of people in Eastern Europe. Those years were kind to Western democracies too. The 'peace dividend' allowed governments to divert budget resources away from defence spending. New consumer markets were opening. There was a glut of low-cost labour in former communist countries with educated workforces, which meant manufacturing costs fell and stuff got cheaper.

This was the benign, temperate global climate – the Great Moderation (described in Chapter 3) – that permitted a flourishing of intellectual complacency at the liberal centre of British politics.

---

* *The End of History and the Last Man*. Fukuyama had first expressed his ideas in an essay three years earlier.

The ride was not always smooth. The age of liberal preening did not exclude shocks. History kept happening. The terrorist attacks on 11 September 2001 were as colossal an event for America's post-war generations as Pearl Harbor had been for their parents and grandparents. In the traumatized aftermath, the menace of jihadi Islamism was often described as existential for the West. But it didn't really shake Western intellectual smugness. Jihadi Islamism was feared for the damage it could inflict, but not as a rival system. It was viewed by secular liberals as a resentful retreat from modernity – retro-medieval barbarism that could only appeal to a minority of malcontents. The terrorists' doctrine might wound democracies and provoke them into illiberal reactions, but it was not a serious ideological rival on the Cold War model.

The 2007–8 financial crisis was a more profound challenge. It offered an irrefutable rebuke to the idea that markets channelled collective wisdom and that state regulation was the enemy of efficient resource distribution. But the scale of government intervention to avert total calamity was treated more as a one-off expedient than a lesson in the perils of ultra-liberal capitalism. In Britain, ideological complacency was suspended only for long enough for the banks to be bailed out, then restored.

If there is any single date on which the post-war period can be said to have ended, it is 24 February 2022, when Russia invaded Ukraine.

It is not the mere fact of war that marked the change. The Balkans had burned in the nineties while the west of the continent congratulated itself on having achieved peace and reconciliation. Nor could it be said that Vladimir Putin's model of government – vintage fascism with a trollish digital extension

– offered a credible rival system to liberal democracy. But the scale of the Russian assault was bigger than anything witnessed in Europe since the early 1940s. And Putin's motive, being the elimination of Ukraine as a nation and its dissolution into a Slavic motherland with Moscow as its capital, was from the same sinister archive.

Those facts alone might not have shaken Western liberals to their ideological core if the core had felt more secure. But the preceding years had witnessed a series of challenges to the institutional architecture of the post-war consensus. A system built to twentieth-century specifications had already come to look rickety and unfit for present challenges. Western solidarity had been rattled by Donald Trump's marauding Europhobic nationalism. European unity had been sabotaged by Brexit. Illiberal nationalists were gobbling chunks of mainstream politics inside the European Union.

China had emerged as a global superpower, nearing parity with the US. It had achieved this by embracing a form of state-directed capitalism without concessions to multi-party democracy – a feat that was not supposed to be possible in the 'end of history' analysis. The theory had been that market freedoms generate affluent middle classes that want their property rights protected and issue irresistible demand for political rights, freedoms and the rule of law.

The post-war world order was meant to be self-reinforcing in a virtuous liberal circle of capitalism and democracy. That complacency, born of economic globalization in the nineties, was then hard-wired into the Western operating system as part of a technological revolution that happened to be kicking off at the same time.

(iii) 'Don't be evil'

In 2000, *Wired* magazine, the leading journal to explore the connection between technology and culture, made an optimistic prognosis about the relationship between the internet and politics:

> We are, as a nation, better educated, more tolerant, and more
> connected because of – not in spite of – the convergence of
> the internet and public life. Partisanship, religion, geography,
> race, gender, and other traditional political divisions are
> giving way to a new standard – wiredness – as an organizing
> principle for political and social attitudes.

The view of interconnectedness as an engine of progress was typical of the time. The spirit of digital enterprise emanating from Silicon Valley was utopian and evangelical. It bundled exuberance in the expectation of commercial profits with idealism in believing that politics would be remade, recoded to be more free.

The theory was that unstoppable information, flowing along millions of autonomous peer-to-peer channels, would bypass the old hierarchies. Dictatorship and repression would be impractical; impossible. Tyrants and censors were artefacts of analogue statecraft that would be made obsolete.

'Governments of the Industrial World, you weary giants of flesh and steel, I come from Cyberspace, the new home of Mind,' wrote the libertarian John Perry Barlow in his 1996 Declaration of the Independence of Cyberspace. 'I declare the global social space we are building to be naturally independent of the tyrannies you seek to impose on us.'

'The Net interprets censorship as damage,' said John Gilmore, co-founder of the Electronic Frontier Foundation, 'and routes around it.' It was widely asserted that no durable partition or enclosure of the new global common land was possible.

The sunniness of that outlook reflected the intellectual climate of the times – the belief that the history train had glided into its liberal terminus – and the climate of Northern California.

It is no coincidence that San Francisco became the hub of the tech boom in the nineties, having previously been the spiritual home of flower power, psychedelic rock and the whole late-sixties Haight-Ashbury stew of anarchists, activists and acid freaks. Seeds of idealism and irreverence were left scattered around the Bay Area long after most of the hippies had gone home. They landed on fertile soil, irrigated by the old pioneer spirit of the California Gold Rush.

The unique fruit that rose a generation later was the Silicon Valley start-up ethos that combined voracious entrepreneurial capitalism with counter-cultural veneration for all things communal. The product was a paradoxical but lucrative hybrid ethos of greed and sharing, and a tech model that evolved uncanny ways of making people very rich by ostensibly giving services out for free. Google felt sufficiently secure in its status as a beneficent force in the universe that it took 'Don't be evil' as a corporate motto (since abandoned).

Techno-optimism peaked at the end of the noughties. There were flashes of political vindication around the world, starting with the Green Movement that sprang up in Iran in the aftermath of a fraudulent presidential election in 2009. Authorities in the Islamic Republic were disoriented by the new, decentralized and spontaneous character of protests that could be called into being by mobile phones. Social media played the same catalytic role in the Arab Spring the following year. The theory that digitization could defeat despots looked sound.

But over a decade later, Iran was still a fundamentalist theocracy. As for the Arab Spring, only Tunisia maintained a shaky democracy, and that was mostly shut down by 2021. Egypt quickly turned autocratic. Libya, Syria and Yemen were consumed by civil war. The internet gave a precious glimpse of political freedom to the victims of those conflicts, but the window was not wide enough for whole nations to make their escape from repression. A vastly increased capacity for information to flow out of war zones did little to inspire sustained compassion in Western audiences.

Cyber-idealism yielded to brutal politics and brute commerce. The internet proved susceptible to censorship and manipulation by thuggish state authorities. China erected its Great Firewall. The billions of people whose lives are most shaped by the legacy of the Tiananmen Square massacre can't even google it. Their Western peers get their kicks on TikTok, owned by ByteDance, headquartered in Beijing.

Declarations of cyber-independence mean nothing to the Chinese Communist Party or Putin. The US tech companies that amassed more collective wealth and influence over a wider dominion than any empire in history did not build democratic safeguards into their products, because that wasn't their business.

Facebook founder Mark Zuckerberg was honest about the hierarchy of information around which his site's moneymaking apparatus would be built when he said: 'A squirrel dying in front of your house may be more relevant to your interests right now than people dying in Africa.' He wasn't wrong. A service designed to satisfy parochial news priorities was never going to focus on mechanisms that might prevent its misuse for the spread of lies and dark propaganda.

In 2018, Facebook admitted that its platform had been an effective tool for the incitement of violence – a genocidal campaign of killings and mass expulsions – against Myanmar's Rohingya minority in previous years. An independent report commissioned by the company found that it had become an 'enabling environment' for the proliferation of human rights abuses.

The Silicon Valley tech utopians were wrong about the vulnerability of authoritarian states to a networked citizenship. They were also blind to the effect in established Western democracies. The theory stated that wiring everyone together would spread the benign liberal ethos that happened to be in the balmy California air when the circuits were designed. The model didn't factor in a change in the climate.

As with previous industrial revolutions, the emerging class of tech magnates didn't anticipate – or didn't care – that their machines would spill toxic waste into public spaces. By the time the effect was too big to ignore, they were rich and powerful enough to lobby against regulations that might force them to clean up the mess.

A conflict between the imperatives of the market and the health of civic democracy had not been in the original manifesto of the digital revolution. It is only now, in the post-post-war climate, that the choice can be seen in such stark terms.

(iv) Mind the gap

Democracy prevailed in 1945 by winning a war, not an argument. Churchill did not debate the Nazis into realizing the error of their ways, and not all of the Allied powers were committed to political freedom in the first place. The Western liberal style of government was spared annihilation and took credit for the victory over fascism, but to say it won because it was the superior system neglects the decisive role of Soviet power. As Clive James put it: 'Whole libraries written to Hitler's detriment didn't add up to the effect of a single Russian artillery shell.'

Eastern Europe had to wait a while for democracy to win the twentieth century.

Even after the Cold War, the picture was muddied by the terms of surrender imposed on the losing side. An Estonian friend who grew up under Soviet occupation once told me that *Dallas* and soft toilet roll did more than dissident literature and demonstrations to bring about the collapse of communism. He meant that a taste for luxuriant Western lifestyles mobilized public frustration as much as the absence of political rights. Estonians could pick up the American soap opera from nearby Finnish TV transmitters, and non-abrasive lavatory paper was smuggled across the water from Helsinki.

Nothing should detract from the bravery of campaigners who stood up to the Communist Party, often with no hope of success. Their struggle laid the moral foundations for victory over dictatorship. But the abject failure of communist economies to deliver improved living standards was the most powerful engine of mass disillusionment.

The demand for freedom encompassed many things. The right to live unmolested by a bullying state and release from the grinding drabness of Soviet anti-consumerism were packaged together. Capitalism and democracy were coupled in the minds of people craving release from communism. They were fused even tighter in the self-esteem of Western politicians who congratulated themselves as the liberators of the East.

In Britain and the US, in particular, the collapse of the Berlin Wall was taken as endorsement of a specific brand of capitalism – the version that saw free markets not just as an adjunct to political liberty, but as the only reliable safeguard of democracy.

The kernel of that argument existed before a Cold War was declared, set out in Friedrich Hayek's 1944 book *The Road to Serfdom*. Hayek, an Austrian economist who fled the Third Reich and later taught in Britain and America, argued that state control of the economy inevitably violated individual agency, leading to denial of personal freedom. In that view, socialism was always antithetical to democracy. The ambition to manage an economy towards more equal outcomes would tend towards totalitarianism. That analysis fitted the Soviet case study, where the line between political repression and economic coercion was blurred. Hayek's theory ossified into dogma when adopted as statecraft by Margaret Thatcher* and Ronald Reagan.

It was demonstrably true that market economies managed through competitive multi-party politics generated wealth and

---

* Veneration of Hayek extends to Thatcher's great admirer Liz Truss, who was a student member of Oxford University's Hayek Society – a club for devotees of markets and individual liberty.

satisfied citizens' needs better than one-party states that tried to allocate resources from an all-powerful central command.

But the next stage in the ideological evolution of anti-socialist thinking was more contestable. It was not proven that the most useful thing a government could do for its citizens was cut their taxes to a minimum, withdraw the provision of services and generally get out of the way. That was where a moral victory for political liberalism (the demand for freedom from oppression) was co-opted to bolster the economic case for neo-liberalism – laissez-faire economics and an automatic presumption that private enterprise would meet society's needs more effectively than the state.*

Successive crises in the early twenty-first century have already furnished ample rebuke to the Thatcherite compulsion to be always shrinking the state (although the lesson has not been quickly heeded). As noted above, the financial crisis made a case for state intervention that was largely neglected by Britain's liberal-conservative coalition government.

Some Tories discerned a rising cry of demand for state protections in the Brexit referendum result. Theresa May arrived in Downing Street, promising to address 'burning injustices' and re-orient her party towards 'the good that government can do'. But her premiership was incinerated by the harm that Brexit did before she got round to that.

Boris Johnson acknowledged the same imperative when he

---

* It's more complicated than that, of course, which is why I'm not a great fan of 'neo-liberalism' as a label. It tends to be used imprecisely as a term of general abuse hurled by the left at anyone who recognizes that capitalism works. But it does describe a genuine movement in the evolution of political economy, and sometimes no other word quite fits the bill.

made 'levelling up' a defining goal of his administration. But the flat-pack slogan was never erected into anything amounting to three-dimensional policy. The pandemic also forced Johnson's government to overturn decades of anti-interventionist conviction, directly subsidizing the wages of millions of workers to keep enterprises alive through lockdowns.

Then came Russia's invasion of Ukraine, with its second front as a war of economic attrition against the West. The Kremlin weaponized gas exports to the rest of Europe. That proved the limits to what a free-market model can achieve when a bloody dictator has his finger on the power switch that feeds the market.

The message appears to have reached the electorate. By 2022, many Conservative voters were telling opinion pollsters that they viewed nationalization of utility companies and transport services favourably, or at least without horror. Events have washed some of the ideological dye of Thatcherism out of the fabric of public opinion, if not from the upper echelons of the Tory party.

Climate change, easily the single greatest political challenge of the foreseeable future, demands strategic state investment and public management of resources on a scale that upsets adherents of neo-liberal economics so much that many of them choose instead to deny that the crisis exists.

By the bleak winter of 2022–3, it was no longer intellectually credible to govern by allergic recoil from government inter-vention, although that was Liz Truss's strongest instinct. In the contest to replace Boris Johnson as Conservative leader, she resisted the idea of a subsidy on fuel bills for struggling households and businesses, declaring there would be 'no handouts'. She ended up committing tens of billions of pounds to the cause of cushioning people against the cold.

Truss venerated the embalmed corpse of her beloved ideology with the pious rigidity of Soviet politburo bosses surveying victory parades from Lenin's marble mausoleum on Red Square. But financial markets are unsentimental about such devotion when the numbers don't add up. The City spurned her September 2022 'mini-budget' – a frenzy of tax cuts with no plan for compensating revenue beyond the hocus-pocus of conjuring growth with enterprising spirits. The pound tanked; the cost of UK debt soared; the government fell.

Rishi Sunak took over with a lament for Truss's mistakes without specifying what they had been. He was installed by the Tories to restore their credibility but not licensed to change their convictions. The gap between the state of the country as most people experienced it and the world as the ruling party declared it to be yawned wider towards grim absurdity.

Britain was slow to recognize that it had reached the end of an ideological road. Partly, that was the numbing effect of the phoney Brexit revolution. Too many people in the political and media class had been complicit in the fraudulent misdirection of national energy into strategic and economic self-harm. Their embarrassment, configured as denial, dulled the clamour for a drastic change of direction.

There was also the stickier residue of that end-of-history spirit that had taught a generation to suppose it lived in a post-ideological age as well as a post-war one. Free-market economics and liberal politics were not contested propositions in the mainstream of election contests at the turn of the twenty-first century. The Tories were only the most capitalist among capitalist parties. The Liberal Democrats struggled to carve out a distinct ideological niche for themselves precisely because the bigger parties also housed liberals and democrats.

For most of the second half of the twentieth century, the case for Western-style governance hardly needed making on its own terms because comparisons with the alternatives – recently remembered fascism and still extant communism – were so eloquent. There was also a happy alignment of political stability and consumer satisfaction. Britain had representative government, human rights and luxury toilet paper. Liberal politics and liberal economics were in sync. There was no pressure to spell out the specific merits of either, or disentangle them, if they worked in tandem.

The economic covenant that underwrites British democracy might be tacit, but that doesn't mean voters are relaxed if it is broken. A vital clause was the promise that each generation would do better than its parents. That stopped happening in the noughties. Median wages in Britain stagnated after 2007, then fell in real terms. In late 2022, living standards were savaged by the return of double-digit inflation – a scourge largely forgotten since the early 1980s. By 2023, real incomes were scarcely higher than they had been 20 years earlier. Productivity gains were nil. The twenty-first century had been an economic hamster wheel for the nation, running ever harder, advancing nowhere.

In Britain, notions of personal and collective economic success are intimately connected to property – owning a home once indicated arrival at maturity as a citizen; the increased value of that home was insulation against future penury. On those metrics, the British economy offers mostly despair to generations born after 2000. The average age of a first-time buyer has been creeping steadily up. The post-war peak for young people acquiring properties was 1989. In that year, 51 per cent of 25–34-year-olds had a foot on the ladder. By 2016, it was half as many.

The millennial generation* and its successors are far more likely than their parents to be renting their homes, using a growing portion of a shrinking income for shelter, with even less left over to stay warm and fed. Those constraints force young people to delay starting families of their own. They must rely on parents or grandparents to subsidize them into adulthood, or be poor if that isn't an option. Most people who are not yet of pension age now face working into their dotage without prospect of retirement income. Vast regional and inter-generational inequalities were a structural feature of the British economy even before soaring energy costs and rising prices sent immiserating shock waves through parts of the country that had presumed themselves to be insulated from poverty.

A society where young people can't afford to have children and increasing numbers of parents struggle to put food on the table for the families they have is facing a crisis of political legitimacy.

All forms of government imply a bargain between rulers and those they rule. The former get power in exchange for providing the latter with security and prosperity. Authoritarian regimes can use coercion to maintain control if they can't uphold their end of the deal. In democracies, the contract is renewed when

---

* Millennials, or Generation Y, are usually identified as those born between 1981 and 1996. A lot changed over that period, which is why generalization about whole cohorts is a horribly blunt tool for any political analysis. Bobby Duffy's book *Generations* is an excellent guide to what is true and what is myth in this field.

there is a change of government. Prolonged breakdown of that mechanism stress-tests public trust in democracy to levels unseen for generations.

Economic hardship needs a cushion of faith that the system is self-correcting. Political turbulence can be severe if it is expected to be temporary. That confidence is harder to sustain in conditions of permacrisis, living on the side of a volcano that erupts again before the last lava flow has cooled.

Market failures, whether in housing, energy or employment, contain a moral as well as a financial challenge to the foundations of post-war capitalist ideology. They break the link between work and progress. The Thatcher–Reagan model presumes automatic and proportionate reward for individual effort. In theory, markets are perfectly meritocratic because talented people outcompete less able rivals. As long as everyone has equal rights at the starting line, success in life is the measurable output derived from your personal input. You are the author of your own destiny, and if your life sucks, you have no one to blame but yourself.

That axiom is no less clumsy in its failure to account for actual human experience than the Marxist analysis in which individual success and failure are understood as expressions of class dynamics. Like Marxism, the free-market theory that wealth accrues to the industrious then trickles down to the rest confuses the desirable with the inevitable. It takes a fantasy of how things *should* work as a description of how they *are*, which relieves governments of the obligation to fix things.

In reality, fair but unfettered competition is no easier to achieve than any other utopian goal. Interventions and corrections will always be needed along the way. There are external forces that interfere to thwart success, misfortunes that money cannot palliate, and deep structural imbalances that make life easier for people born in certain families, to certain kinds (and colours) of parent.

Even if you could somehow measure and correct all of those imbalances, the meritocratic promise would still be a lie. There is a problem that the philosopher Michael Sandel identifies in his 2020 book *The Tyranny of Merit*: even a relatively egalitarian model will struggle to eliminate differential status, which means some jobs will be better paid and have greater social cachet than others.

A higher minimum wage can put food on the table of people who sweep streets, stack shelves or work in call centres. Unemployment benefits can support those who have no job. But welfare and tax credits can't remove the stigma of a lowly condition in the social pecking order; especially not when the system is arranged around the idea that low status is the deserved outcome of your individual choices.

That ethos is tolerable for as long as enough people who feel they have worked hard, played by the rules and done everything that was asked of them earn enough to heat their homes and feed themselves. If they can't, they would rather not be told it is their fault. Politics will then become a competition to find alternative explanations for their misfortune.

Nationalism is on hand to denounce the usual scapegoats – foreigners and their cosmopolitan accomplices. There will always be an audience for that message, but it doesn't have to be the dominant strain of British politics.

Other stories are available. There are appeals to collective solidarity, moderation and mutual tolerance that have deep roots in British culture and a purchase on national identity. It is not hard to imagine a future where those values are more attractive than the shrivelled, sour husk of an ideology that can imagine progress only as the aggregation of every individual's merciless self-interest.

It is not always easy to tell the difference between the putrescence of a long-incumbent regime and the obsolescence of policies enacted by that government. Within weeks of its formation, Liz Truss's government displayed signs of both. She and her Chancellor, Kwasi Kwarteng, hurtled into libertarian dogma with such intemperate haste that the markets they claimed to venerate spat out their growth plan in disgust. Neither Kwarteng nor Truss were unintelligent people, but they took ideological stupefaction to its most extreme level as zombification – the point where a doctrine begins to feast on its own rotten flesh.

The fate of that short-lived administration cannot contain a full audit of what is living and what needs burying from the late-twentieth-century model of free-market capitalism. Truss's attachment to the theory had the monomaniac intensity of a cult, which made it hard to know what portion might have been viable in less fanatical hands.

When Rishi Sunak took over, he sought to compensate for Truss's libertarian excess with budget discipline. The cost of economic and political failure would be felt most acutely by people who depended most on state services and benefits; the resentment fomented by degrading the public realm would be addressed with blame-shifting, culture war and diversion. The Conservative grievance machine turned full circle, back to where it had begun twelve years earlier when David Cameron entered Downing Street and started pandering to the Faragist tendency on his back benches. Britain had squandered a dozen years on a pointless crusade incited by nationalist zealots to a holy land that didn't exist to fight enemies who were really friends, defeating no one but itself.

Locked in a cycle of stagnation and convulsive crisis, British democracy has struggled to honour its traditional economic promise to voters. That failure doesn't yet resemble the depth of ideological decay that hollowed out the Soviet bloc. Not yet, but there are disturbing likenesses.

There is a disparity between the ambitions that give our system its defining purpose and the reality experienced by people whose consent is needed to keep the system going. It is a gap that could make the whole system look like a sham. If the gap is not closed, the ideology comes to look like an organized hypocrisy; a game that serves the elite while pretending to deliver a growing bounty for the masses. Those are conditions in which the Potemkin syndrome flourishes – hypercynicism, despairing disengagement, conspiracy theory and rage breaking out as the sweat on democracy's fevered brow.

(v) The centre holds

What is the shelf life of a political system? It is now more than three decades since the collapse of the Soviet Union. The Berlin Wall has been down longer than it was ever up, which is long enough for a Western model that was once flexible and vigorous to look stale and sclerotic. That doesn't mean it is doomed. But it suggests that renewal cannot be achieved simply by yanking harder on rusty old policy levers.

An essential division in politics is now between those who are meaningfully engaged with the scale of the challenge and those who are too stupefied by ideology to grasp what is at stake. When founding principles of the democracy need reaffirming, the boundary that matters most is between those who can be candid in admitting the nature of the task and charlatans whose stock in trade is simplicity and blame.

In the first chapter of this book, I identified a basic function of democratic politics as peaceful mediation between conflicting social interests. I went on to describe the ways that populism and nationalism discredit a representative democratic system by denying the existence of those conflicts, exacerbating the tensions that arise from them, sowing division in the name of unity.

In Part Two, I looked at the underlying strains on democracy that help generate the demand for populist and nationalist politics – the unhealthy symptoms of insecurity, polarization, mistrust and radicalization that militate against compromise, nuance and conciliation.

In Part Three, I described the conditions that led to a revolution against centrist politics, and the bogus character of that revolution – how it hijacked social and economic frustration that had been building for generations; how a self-serving revolutionary elite locked itself onto a course of vandalism in the name of renewal; how the inevitable failure of that approach would lead to a cynical politics of stoking the grievances that outmoded ideological prescriptions could never resolve.

It will not be easy to get politics out of that rut. Denial of the problem is carved into its contours. Restoring healthy function to British democracy begins with a recognition that governing is hard; that the tasks are complex; that there are trade-offs and unavoidable compromises. That message can sound uninspiring, unambitious and bleak, but it needn't always be so. There is an opportunity in the failure of nationalist and populist government to make the principled case for pragmatism. There is an idealistic argument for non-ideological government. When doctrinaire leaders are mired in chaos, ordinary competence is illuminated as a rare leadership virtue.

In the peak period of liberal complacency, the argument for moderation as a moral choice went unrehearsed. The foundation of that case is the reliable tendency of radicals to fail and then defend their failure with bullying and lies. In the mid-twentieth century, when the historical proof of that proposition was recent, the argument made itself. Now it needs to be remade, and there is a fresh store of evidence at home and abroad to support it.

The location of that political revival can still be called the centre ground. That has felt like a sparsely populated zone in recent years, but the cacophony of maniacs should not be mistaken for proof that they are the majority. As noted in Chapter 6, a throng of noisy extremists at either end of the spectrum drowns out a mass of quieter opinion in the middle.

In Chapter 10, I observed how centrism came to be despised by radicals of left and right as the meretricious code of Westminster courtiers. Puritan ideologues suspect centrists of pawning their party's soul for the votes of unbelievers. That judgement was bolstered by a succession of ballots – the Brexit referendum, the 2017 and 2019 general elections – that made the old liberal centre ground look infertile as electoral terrain.

But there is a distinction to be drawn between the fixed

geometry of centrist politics as defined at the turn of the century and centrism as an ethos that prefers persuasion and evidence to dogma and denunciation.

One common charge against middle-way politics is that it preaches cowardly satisfaction with least-worst outcomes when courage in conviction would deliver better ones. Another is that the adaptation to majority opinion risks complicity in wickedness when extreme ideas have permeated the mainstream. That threat is not negligible. There is such a thing as a compromise too far. But the risk is also exaggerated by people who draw the line as a tight boundary around their own narrow political prejudice.

A centrist prospectus cannot chart a third way between populist fantasies and governing realities. It has to side with the latter, but that is not a niche position. Reality is where most people dwell, most of the time.

Nor can a new centrism be a mere tribute act to the liberal consensus that dominated the late twentieth century. The task is to rehabilitate a moderating and pragmatic instinct that was misplaced in the frenzy of hubris at the misdiagnosed end of history; then apply it in the new landscape as shaped by history's vengeance.

Some parameters have not changed. In economic policy, the extreme bounds of left and right are where they always were. Monolithic state control is an affront to liberty. But floating all human fortunes on the market leads to atrocious inequality. There is a vast spectrum of available opinion between those poles. It is possible to believe that private commerce and the profit motive drive prosperity while recognizing also that under-regulation and the retreat of government from the provision of essential services breed dissatisfaction that leads to instability.

The same is true of a cultural spectrum ranging between liberal and conservative perspectives on national identity. It is possible to believe that respect for tradition is a ballast that stabilizes a society in tumultuous times; also that the historical record is open to reinterpretation by new generations with changed values – and that there are patriots on both sides of that proposition.

Recognizing that an alternative perspective is valid in principle doesn't have to blend politics into consensual mush. There are acres of ground for impassioned disagreement on every policy, from raising taxes to pulling down statues, while staying within the bounds of liberal democracy. There are not many things that parties must all agree on, but consensus on some foundational principles of democracy is vital. As a starting point, rivals in any debate or campaign must reject the view of politics as a zero-sum game in which the prize for victory is an opportunity to rig the system so power might never be surrendered again.

Parties will always have ideological components, just as they will always contain utopian idealists. But those tendencies need their counterweight in wariness of zealots and a preference for evidence over faith as the foundation of belief. Leaders who purge pragmatists will soon forfeit their licence to govern.

There is no harm in having steadfast beliefs. The danger comes when opinions are held with such intensity that criticism is construed as treason and reasonable challenge denounced as heresy.

One possible exception, a belief worth holding sacred, is the conviction that democracy itself is a superior form of government to the alternatives. That view doesn't preclude the free expression of anti-democratic ideas, which can be tolerated in confidence that they will fail.

But how strong is that confidence? It has been misplaced before. History proves that democracy is better than dictatorship, but that is a reason why it *should* survive, not a guarantee that it will. The crises of recent years give cause for both optimism and pessimism on that score. Finding the right balance, treading the line between complacency and despair, can be wearying, demoralizing. At every turn there is a temptation to disengage, to follow the sheltered path of internal emigration. This, for me, has been the biggest challenge – politically, psychologically, emotionally.

That is why I have put it off until the last chapter.

CHAPTER 14

THE PARADOX OF VIGILANCE

We never fall into the same abyss twice. But we fall in the same way,
in a mixture of ridicule and dread.

Eric Vuillard

(i) The teeth of Oświęcim

Oświęcim is cold in the first week of November, exposed in the
middle of the Polish plain, bitten by wind and swept by frost.
Wear sturdy shoes, we were told by the organizer of our trip,
and a hat, gloves. Most of the time you will be outdoors. There
will be much walking. I heeded the warning but didn't need to
be told. I had done my share of winters in Eastern Europe. The
guidance was for the benefit of the schoolchildren, sixth-form
history students mostly, who made up the majority of our party.
There were also a couple of other journalists and two MPs, one
Labour, one Tory.

Just as I had thought the weather would hold no surprises for
me, I expected to learn little from Oświęcim that I didn't already
know from the books I had read, films I had seen, stories handed
down in childhood. Although in every previous citation, the little
Polish town had been known by its German name: Auschwitz.

We visited the pre-war Jewish cemetery, or what was left of it. The gravestones had been ripped up during the Nazi era and used to pave streets. Then we visited the first prison site, the constellation of brick buildings that is entered by way of an iron gate over which there still stands the wrought legend *Arbeit Macht Frei*; work makes you free.

Our guide took us through the history and evolution of the camp, including the house where the commandant lived; the garden where his children played. He explained how the infrastructure was unequal to the growing volume of prisoners and how the crematoria could not cope with the mounting pile of corpses. We boarded our coach and moved on to the expansion site that was built to accommodate the camp's surging population of inmates – and the logistical pressure to dispose of them – after 1942, as the Reich's population of Jews and other undesirables was 'resettled' to the East.

I knew this already. I knew about the sealed trains and the sifting process that happened on the platform straight after arrival; how doctors discerned who was capable of work and sent the rest to extermination. I knew about the pegs on which the victims were instructed to hang their coats, and how they were told to remember the location because they would be back to collect their items after a shower. I knew that the shower heads dispensed Zyklon B – cyanide gas. I knew about the mountain of round-rimmed spectacles and the rolls of fabric woven from human hair. Nothing was casually discarded by the camp administration, apart from humanity.

As the sun went down and the freezing wind picked up, our guide led us to the remains of one of the gas chambers. When Allied forces closed in, the Nazis tried to destroy the evidence by blowing up the rooms used for slaughter. Here was a place where the testimony stops, because none who entered survived. There can be no knowledge of what happened there without a leap of imagination, and imagination flinches from the drop.

But I had not known about the teeth.

The gas chambers and crematoria were operated by the *Sonderkommando*, 'special units' under SS command but recruited from camp inmates, usually in that first selection straight after disembarkation. It is normal practice in any penal colony to enlist prisoners to the machinery of repression. It sows division, breaks spirits and spares valued officers and men from the dirtiest work. History knows few jobs dirtier. It wouldn't be entirely right to say they had no choice. There were cases of refusal to comply, followed by immediate execution. Those who did comply were not spared, but they were allowed to live for the duration of their complicity. Testimony from the *Sonderkommando* is fragmentary. Notes were hidden around the site. There is a memoir; some blurred photographs. And there are teeth, which withstand the oven temperature that incinerates flesh. The prisoners tasked with disposing of the ashes picked out the surviving teeth and buried them in the field next to the gas chambers.

In *The Drowned and the Saved*, Primo Levi dedicates several pages to the *Sonderkommando* in a chapter entitled 'The Grey Zone'. In it, he confronts the moral problem posed when crime and victim are contained in the same person. He brings a magnifying lens to the darkest part of human experience to show how, even in the place where right and wrong should be clearly delineated, even in Auschwitz, there can still be an intersection where the two spheres meet. Levi does not say this to excuse any Nazis. He is clear in his refusal to indulge the defence that the murderers were only obeying orders, which would be to 'confuse them with their victims'. It is true that systematic atrocity damages the perpetrators, too, and that many are later tormented by their actions, but the harms belong in different categories. Torturer and tortured are not interchangeable roles.

Levi's point is to illustrate that our need to make sense of the world, and thereby live in it with some mental equilibrium, involves moral pattern-finding. That process approximates truth and obscures some of it in the process: 'What we commonly mean by "understand" coincides with "simplify": without profound simplification the world around us would be an infinite, undefined tangle that would defy our ability to orient ourselves and decide upon our actions.'

There is no point denying the simplifying urge. It is ancient and constant. Arranging the world into winners and losers, heroes and villains, righteous and wicked is as natural and automatic when navigating social and political environments as it is necessary to have left, right, up and down to describe positions in physical landscapes. But as Levi argues, recognizing that the reductive trait is human doesn't mean we have to accept moral approximations as definitive: 'This *desire* for simplification is justified, but the same does not always apply to the simplification itself. It is a working hypothesis, useful so long as it is recognized as such and not mistaken for reality.'

Levi's grey zone poses a challenge when trying to measure the scale of a threat to democracy. It would be convenient if the enemy always arrived in uniform and the edge of the abyss were clearly signposted. But it isn't like that in real life.

When I was consumed by fury at the state of British politics, the affliction contained two contradictory emotions. One was dread at how bad things might get. The other was irritation at the casual invocation of worst-case scenarios – the threat of fascism or Stalinism resurgent – to score easy political points. I was afraid of the abyss and angry that fear of the abyss was being cheapened.

When I was growing up, the Holocaust reached out from history to rebuke anyone who thought it was only history. It had a timeless moral dimension that transcended local context and individual circumstance. It was not an argument that started 'on the one hand', because there was no other hand. In political debate on all topics there are layers of motive to peel back. You can drill down into the reasons why people act as they do, examining both sides of a question, weighing the choices someone might make to vote this way or that, fight or surrender. But the collective memory of evil, and the inadequacy of any milder word to convey the character of Nazi Germany, felt to me like a bedrock of intuitive justice beneath which no mitigation could be excavated. The question was not whether absolute categories of right and wrong existed, but whether you – whether I – might recognize the moment to choose between them when it came.

History might look back and see a threshold where equivocation became complicity. But is that threshold visible in the present? Would we know it was there if we had already crossed it?

Anyone who tries to imagine how they might react if the worst were to happen – under military occupation, or if democracy crumbled – is probably searching for interior reassurance that they would be with the resistance. It isn't likely, from a statistical perspective. Judging by the record of how occupied populations tend to behave, most of us would end up collaborating one way or another.

I once interviewed Colette Marin-Catherine, a veteran of the French resistance to Nazi occupation who became the star of an Oscar-winning short film. It shows how she overcame a lifelong aversion to treading on German soil, accompanying a young historian to the site of the concentration camp where her brother, also a resistance fighter, had died in slave labour. She was 92 years old when we met, slight but not frail. Her speech was slow, deliberate, like a sequence of stones thrown into water.

I was interested in her decision to join the resistance, but Colette refused to see it as a choice. She described it as a role she ended up in because it was the obvious thing to do under the circumstances. She took the same view of compatriots who had collaborated. Most of them were just doing what seemed natural. 'It was because they were hungry,' she said. For others it was about keeping a business going, a way to carry on normal life in the groove that events were carving out in front of them. 'They had nothing else to do. It was an activity, like any other activity.'

If the Battle of Britain had been lost, the nation would have adapted to German rule. There were enough politicians who had supported the pre-war policy of appeasement to staff a puppet administration. Nazi race policy had no quarrel with Anglo-Saxon types, so non-Jews would have been unmolested as long as they didn't resist.*

---

* Before the war, much of the Establishment saw a more imminent threat to its interests in Bolshevism, to which Hitler was conveniently opposed. The fate of Jews was, at most, a second-order question. In English aristocratic circles, where a genteel anti-Semitism prevailed, the Nazi version was considered vulgar in its excess but not wrong in its analysis.

On the portion of British territory that *was* occupied – the Channel Islands – the pattern of compliance was much as it was elsewhere in Europe. There was also an active fifth column of Nazi sympathizers on the mainland, itching to commit acts of sabotage. They were identified by MI5 and tricked into collaboration with a fake Gestapo agent, who collected the intelligence they thought they were passing on to the Reich and filed it safely in Whitehall. At the end of the war, a decision was made not to prosecute that hidden battalion of traitors, largely because it would have been embarrassing. Their existence contradicted the story Britain wanted to tell itself about its unflinching resistance to evil.

Most of the time, most people get on with their lives and adapt to political circumstance. The point at which it is morally imperative to choose the path of self-sacrifice might already be in the past, so why martyr yourself for a lost cause? And it is rarely just self-sacrifice. What if the decision to resist puts friends and family in danger? What if the choice to collaborate affords occasions for small acts of mercy along the way? There is a lot of grey zone.

The easy part of vigilance is looking back on past horrors and swearing never to repeat them. The harder part is imagining horrors of the future.

In August 1914, Henry James wrote a letter to his friend and fellow novelist Rhoda Broughton, in which he anticipated the character of a war that most of their contemporaries confidently predicted would be over by Christmas:

> Black and hideous to me is the tragedy that gathers, and I'm
> sick beyond cure to have lived on to see it. You and I, the

ornaments of our generation, should have been spared this
wreck of our belief that through the long years we had seen
civilization grow and the worst become impossible. The tide
that bore us along was then all the while moving to this grand
Niagara – yet what a blessing we didn't know it. It seems to
me to undo everything, everything that was ours, in the most
horrible retroactive way.

I have often wondered about those inflection points when the
arc of history bent away from justice, and progress went into
reverse. Some, like James, could see it happening. Others
retreated into denial or simply weren't paying enough attention.
In Europe in the 1930s, there were people who cowered at the
sight of apocalyptic clouds on the horizon, while others carried
on as usual, their casual gait undisturbed by the drumbeat of
bloodthirsty dictators.

For supporters of appeasement, a duty to avoid repeating
the carnage of the First World War put an ethical gloss on the
misguided policy of trying to bribe Hitler out of starting a
second one.

Prescience was also lacking at the other end of the political
spectrum. Throughout the thirties, left-wing intellectuals visited
Moscow and reported back that communism was delivering on
its utopian promises. In 1934, the novelist H. G. Wells, a
dedicated socialist, interviewed Stalin for the *New Statesman*
and found him 'fair, candid and honest'. The author admitted
that he was unable to judge the full extent of progress, having
only just arrived in the USSR, but 'the happy faces of healthy
men and women' proved that 'something very considerable is
being done here.'

In 1938, *Homes and Gardens* magazine published an enthusiastic tour of Hitler's Bavarian mountain chalet. 'The Führer is his own decorator, designer and furnisher, as well as architect,' the article noted. He also 'has a passion about cut flowers in his home' and 'delights in the society of brilliant foreigners, especially painters, musicians and singers. As host he is a droll raconteur.'

(ii) Waxworks and wolves

The memory of pre-war complacency about the first rise of totalitarianism is supposed to be Western liberal democracy's inoculation against a comeback. Vigilance means staying alert to early indications of the threat. But when aggressive nationalism resurged through Europe and the US, political immune systems did not generate sufficient antibodies to shut it down.

Vladimir Putin's campaign to assert a Greater Russian sovereignty over territory lost when the Soviet Union collapsed was as precisely analogous to Hitler's designs on the Rhineland and Sudetenland as it could have been. The Russian president sounded like a fascist and worked his way through the fascist playbook with methodical predictability. When he launched his all-out assault on Ukraine, many Western leaders were shocked to learn that he meant what he had been saying all along.

A similar combination of naivety and historical amnesia helped propel Donald Trump into the White House. He campaigned as a nationalist demagogue. His flagship policies were explicitly racist. He was endorsed by white supremacists with flaming torches. It was not hard to anticipate that he posed a threat to the liberal constitutional order of the American republic. But conservatives on both sides of the Atlantic strived to convince themselves that it was a kind of arch, knowing performance; as if no one who was an actual fascist would be clumsy enough to behave in such a transparently fascist way.

On the morning after Trump's victory in the November 2016 US presidential election, I was walking through the parliamentary estate, feeling miserable. A Conservative MP (later to become a senior figure in Liz Truss's cabinet) caught my eye. We had spoken many times before, rarely in agreement but always amiably. He was visibly entertained by my glum demeanour. 'You bed-wetting liberals are panicking over nothing,' he said breezily. 'You'll see. He'll govern like an Eisenhower-style Republican.'

To mark Trump's inauguration, *The Times* published a sycophantic interview, conducted not by a staff journalist but by the veteran Tory minister Michael Gove, accompanied by the newspaper's proprietor, Rupert Murdoch. Gove compared Trump's vilification in Britain to the underestimation of George Washington before the American Revolution. He compared the incoming president also to Abraham Lincoln and Ronald Reagan, reporting on Trump's 'warm and genial' demeanour and his 'businessman's ability to cut through jargon to get to the essentials of a case'. Although he could not pretend that the president was an intellectual titan, he was consoled by the recognition that 'intelligence takes many forms.' Perhaps he was also a droll raconteur.

Conceding the extent of Trump's vileness was awkward for British Eurosceptics, who had relished his enthusiasm for Brexit. The Tories were determined to believe that America was immune to fascism, and applied themselves to the task of weaving sheep's clothing for a wolf in the White House who showed no interest in modelling that look.

Far-right paramilitary posses still have a purchase on mainstream opinion in the Republican Party. Trump looked temperamentally amenable to the idea of racist dictatorship. It might have been just a stroke of luck that he was too stupid or disorganized to make it happen. Or it might have been that the constitutional order was resilient. Would it withstand a second assault, led perhaps by a more competent tyrant?

The danger of American democracy collapsing in our lifetime is not negligible. Former neo-Nazi groups have some purchase on the political mainstream in many European countries. An Italian party with fascist roots won a parliamentary election in September 2022. The next president of France might well come from the far right. We do not need to wait for a more precise re-enactment of the 1930s to conclude that vaccination engineered from memories of that time is wearing off.

Sight of what lies at the bottom of the totalitarian abyss is the deterrent against leaping in again. But the force of that argument depends on a clear view of the fall. It fades with time and distance. There are fewer living witnesses, and their vivid testimony has been crowded out by sanitized fiction and lazy hyperbole.

The spectre of a worst-case scenario has become a cliché. For much of my adult life, the most common sighting of Nazis was in the cinema or on TV, as pantomime villains whenever the plot needed an efficient invocation of unalloyed evil.

In politics, reference to fascism became a rhetorical shortcut to moral urgency – a verbal tool for shunting any opponent to the bottom of some slippery hypothetical slope. The radical left will find reason to call any Conservative candidate (and some moderate Labour politicians) fascist. The radical right is as quick on the draw with silly analogy. Tory Eurosceptics have compared the European Union to both the USSR and the Third Reich for wanting to organize the continent into some kind of federalized bloc.

At the height of the pandemic, lockdowns were routinely described by critics of the policy as 'house arrest'. In a radio discussion about a requirement for people to prove their vaccination status, a Conservative MP, Marcus Fysh, objected on the grounds that 'we are not a "papers please" society; this is not Nazi Germany; it's the thin end of an authoritarian wedge.'

Anti-vaccination protesters compared their predicament to the status of Jews in the Third Reich, wearing yellow stars as emblems of their alleged persecution. Women's rights are policed by 'feminazis', in the lexicon of radicalized masculine self-pity. Environmentalists are denigrated by climate science deniers for their 'eco-fascism'.

Decades of casual misuse flipped vigilance into its opposite. Treating 'fascist' as a synonym for whatever you are against, regardless of where you happen to be standing, turns an absolute moral judgement into a relative one, or just a term of abuse. There was such a frenzy of crying wolf that even when the real thing loped into the White House, there was disbelief, coupled with confidence that it could be tamed or that its fangs were just for show.

This is a paradox of vigilance. The determination never to forget was so compulsive that remembering became a mantra, which by mindless repetition bred amnesiac complacency.

The traumas of the twentieth century were preserved, but their power to shock waned. They were installed in what the historian Tony Judt called 'a moral memory palace: a pedagogically serviceable Chamber of Historical Horrors'. The lessons were not entirely forgotten. They were made so universal that everyone thought they could be the teacher and someone else had the duty to learn. The threat was called out everywhere, except the one place where history tells us to be most vigilant of all – in the mirror.

(iii) The wet bias

When the Black Death ravaged Europe in the fourteenth century, troupes of flagellants went from town to town, surrounding local churches, beating themselves with spiky iron-tipped leather scourges. They saw the disease as divine punishment and prayed fervently for release from its clutches, all the while aiding its dispersal across the land. The medical treatments they needed were nearly 600 years away.

Before 2020, a global pandemic had been dreaded by health policy planners and science fiction writers alike as the kind of cataclysm that ends civilization. Then we had one, and within a year there was a vaccine. That isn't to belittle the suffering caused by COVID. The distress was epic and, for millions of people, it is ongoing. But comparison with most plagues in most of recorded history tells a parable of progress. Science was the hero of the tale, and it defeated lies and superstition. Fear that all of politics had become a post-truth bog where facts are submerged in populist sludge turned out to be premature. The bog is still there, but there is also high and firm ground where policy can consort with evidence and data.

It can be hard to take an optimistic view when loitering in the waxwork museum of historical monsters, where the record of good news is not prominently displayed.

Media commentators are especially prone to pessimism, for the same reason that TV meteorologists exhibit a 'wet bias' – exaggerating the probability of rain because audiences are more forgiving of forecasting error in that direction. The umbrella taken but never needed is not resented in the same way as the picnic ruined by an unexpected downpour. The economist whose predicted downturn never materializes is not ridiculed as much as the Pollyanna who bets on an ever bigger boom on the eve of a bust.

I have learned from years of writing a newspaper column that it is easier to imagine everything going wrong than to chart the hypothetical course by which it all turns out for the best. A bet on human frailty and plans coming unstuck is safe. But the hedging bet on human ingenuity finding a way through and most things ticking along fine – and incrementally upwards – is usually underpriced.

In *The Future Starts Here: Adventures in the Twenty-First Century*, John Higgs describes the tendency of Western culture to narrate the present as if the slide into a dystopian future is inevitable, even if the process by which we get there is unclear. It is, he writes, like 'a crime novel with the last page ripped out . . . We don't know exactly the identity of the murderer, but we do know that the story is about to come to an end.'

And yet, as he notes, things routinely defy an intellectual consensus that they will end badly by getting better instead.

Humans are too flawed to make utopias work, but smart enough to dodge dystopias, too.

Giddy optimism and its opposite thrive at times of technological upheaval. Clever machines tend to occupy one of two slots in the human imagination – liberator or jailer; delivering progress or crushing souls. Information technology is especially disorienting because the very thing it promises to replace first – old media – is also the tool we have come to rely on when navigating our way in the world.

The science fiction writer Douglas Adams had three rules to describe generational adaptation to technology:

1. Anything that is in the world when you're born is normal and ordinary and is just a natural part of the way the world works.
2. Anything that's invented between when you're 15 and 35 is new and exciting and revolutionary and you can probably get a career in it.
3. Anything invented after you're 35 is against the natural order of things.

Portable devices are especially prone to induce moral panic in parents, who find it harder to police the flow of information into impressionable young minds. That was as true of the transistor radio blaring out rock 'n' roll in the 1950s as it is for the iPhone that I fail to prise from my children's hands. I urge them to read more novels, which were once also denounced for degrading attention spans and demoralizing readers by presenting unattainable ideals for impossible emulation.

In 1817, the *Gentleman's Magazine*, a periodical digest of essays on matters of social and cultural note, published a warning against 'Novel Reading, a Cause of Female Depravity' that is not far removed from twenty-first-century gripes about Instagram.*

> Those who first made novel-reading an indispensable branch in forming the minds of young women have a great deal to answer for. Without this poison instilled, as it were, into the blood, females in ordinary life would never have been so much the slaves of vice. The plain food, wholesome air, and exercise they enjoy, would have exempted them from the tyranny of lawless passion.

Print was still in relative infancy when readers started complaining about information overload. In 1600, Barnabe Riche, an English author, described the 'multitude of books' as 'one of the great diseases of this age' that 'doth so overcharge the world that it is not able to digest the abundance of idle matter that is every day hatched'. In 1628, Robert Burton, author of a huge treatise on depression, complained that the world was oppressed by the

---

* There does appear to be a case against social media where young people's mental health is concerned. In 2021, a Facebook whistle-blower, Frances Haugen, reported that the company's own private research confirmed what many parents and psychologists already suspected – that teenage girls in particular found Instagram (owned by Facebook) an aggravating factor when they suffered from low self-esteem and anxiety about their bodies. There is evidence that heavy social media use is more widely correlated with depression, but that is as likely to be a symptom as a cause. It makes sense that depressed people would prefer socializing behind a digital cloak of anonymity. That does not prove that consuming online content is what made them depressed in the first place. And having a virtual place to go when analogue interaction feels too much is also a potential source of comfort.

'vast chaos and confusion of books' that made 'our eyes ache with reading, our fingers with turning'.

In 2001, Marc Prensky, an education specialist, published an article on the effect of new technology in education, noting the cross-generational divide between analogue-trained teachers and tech-savvy kids. He compared it to the divide between parents who have moved to a new country and their children who are raised there, immersed in its culture from an early age.

In Prensky's scheme, I am a digital immigrant and my children are digital natives. In the barrier between us I see reflected obstacles I once encountered trying to communicate with my South African parents, whose conditioning in how the world worked sometimes felt thousands of miles out of sync with my experience of childhood. No matter how hard I work at assimilation, I will never speak internet as fluently as the younger generation, and I will never shake the nagging feeling of discomfort at a forsaken homeland where things were easier, simpler, slower.

Digital immigrants are analogue exiles. We find comfort in romantic tales of the old country. Remember how we were all more *present* in the room, not fidgeting with phones? And how we made arrangements in advance and stuck to them? Weren't those drizzly afternoons spent watching sheepdog trials on TV* character-building? Boredom stimulated the imagination and made us better people, right?

---

* For the benefit of younger readers: this was a real thing. At its peak in the early 1980s, *One Man and His Dog* attracted up to eight million viewers (though maybe attracted is the wrong word there, if I was counted in that number).

The underlying argument is that constraint was liberating. Narrower bandwidth broadened horizons. But did it really? Were we any richer for having poorer access to information? Were we more socially adjusted with fewer channels, or just more easily coerced into conformity? One way to answer the question is to consider how readily you would go back.

Politicians and journalists might be exhausted by the relentless pace of news. But it doesn't follow that democracy was healthier when less of it was visible, information was controlled by fewer people drawn from a narrower social cadre and voters were kept at a more respectful distance from power.

I noted in Chapter 6 that polarization and invective date back a lot further than the internet. Culture wars are vile but still preferable to real wars, which for hundreds of years were the standard way to settle differences between implacably opposed tribal identities.

The fear that politics is undermining the foundations of truth is also old. The Scottish writer John Arbuthnot expressed that fear in his 'Art of Political Lying' (not a book itself, but a satirical review imagining such a book) in 1713.

Fake news was around before Facebook. It was the staple of many publications in the nineteenth century, where no attempt was made to distinguish fiction from recorded events. In 1844, the New York *Sun* published a story about a transatlantic hot-air-balloon journey that was an invention of Edgar Allan Poe.

There aren't many technological advances in history that humanity would wish to forget. It is easy to think of undesirable *applications* of technology – nuclear weapons spring to mind – but harder to argue that the underlying knowledge should be expunged from collective consciousness. Also, pointless. There is no going back, and the precedents do not look great in those periods of history when knowledge went astray. What little is known about life in the early-medieval Dark Ages doesn't invite replication.

I have a strong bias in this argument, being alive today only because of scientific innovation. I had the same heart attack as my grandfather at the same age, but he had no mobile phone to call for help, and even if he had done, there were no stents to prop his arteries open.

When technology is shaking up the way we are used to doing things, it is easy to forget that our way is the product of previous shake-ups. The end of the world *as we know it* is not the end of the world. Prophecy of doom is a symptom of volatility in the present, not proof that the future will be worse.

'By the year 2000, the United Kingdom will simply be a small group of impoverished islands, inhabited by some 70 million hungry people.' That was a prediction from 1969 by Paul Ehrlich, an American biologist who became fixated on the threat of excessive population growth. (On that gloomy terrain he was following in the footsteps of Thomas Malthus, the English cleric and economist of the eighteenth century who saw the increasing volume of people in the world as a natural check on progress, which would vanish into the hungry mouths of the ever-renewing horde of needy people.) For Ehrlich, there was the additional threat of nuclear war, which significantly tipped the odds away from future prosperity. 'If I were a gambler, I would take even money that England will not exist in the year 2000.'

Equivalent forecasts of calamity have been published in every decade since the Second World War, usually with re-enactment of that conflict as the plughole down which events will inexorably swirl.

Every generation glimpses but never reaches the collapse of Western democracy. The demise is forecast with relish by radicals and revolutionaries, who plan to build a better society on liberalism's grave. That spooks the moderates and prag-matists, who worry that the utopian extremists have more attractive slogans.

But the long-term trend of human evolution irrefutably tracks a movement away from endemic violence and towards peaceful coexistence. That isn't to say the movement always goes from darkness to light, or from superstition to reason. There is plenty of traffic the other way. But the balance sheet, read across a long enough timeline, is net positive for progress.

A thought experiment: you face being reincarnated at some time in the past with no control over the place or status of your rebirth. You might appear on any continent, in any family, as royalty or in rags. Alternatively, instead of spinning that roulette wheel of history, you can choose to be reborn, also in a random location, but in the present. Which fate do you choose?

On a basic calculus of survival, running the laws of prob-ability, today is by far the safer choice. Any previous time and there is a significant risk of dying on day one. And not great odds on making it past the age of five. If you get beyond child-hood, the prospect of a horrible death by war, famine or disease is way higher for any period in the past compared to now.

Another thought experiment, created by the economist Max Roser: imagine a newspaper that is published once every 50 years. On that cycle, the news looks a lot rosier than it does when churned out daily, or hourly, or every second on Twitter. Items in the most recent edition might include drastic rises in global living standards (around 1 in 10 people on earth live in poverty today compared to 6 in 10 in the middle of the twentieth century); the elimination of smallpox; the availability of food and education to billions of people who used to lack both. The news is not all good, of course. Climate change and collapsing biodiversity cloud the horizon, but even there it is feasible that progress will prevail. In Britain, concern about the environment has leapt from the margins to the mainstream in a relatively short time. It used to animate only younger generations; now it is much more evenly distributed. Denial of the basic science behind global warming persists, but it is much less often given parity with reality in political debate. There will always be sightings of egregious idiocy in the media, but compared to a hyperactive rolling news service, where *everything* looks bleak, the 50-year edition gives cause for comfort.

The historical record doesn't eliminate reasons to worry about the future, but nor does it insist on demoralized panic.

(iv) In the end, the truth wins

In 1914, Europe charged merrily at the abyss, high on technological progress, economic globalization and self-congratulatory modernism. The mechanized slaughter that followed was so horrendous that people imagined nothing like it could happen again. It was a 'war to end war'.* Until the next one. Even if

---

* The phrase was originally coined by H. G. Wells, whose judgement on how war might be eliminated was proved faulty by the conviction that Stalin might be part of the solution.

optimism is justified in the long view of history, the record is particularly cruel to the optimists who call it wrong.

In 1930, a forecast that most of Europe would be better off and peaceful in 30 years' time would be right, but not useful as an account of the near future, given the dark route by which peace and prosperity were reached.

If you zoom the lens of time out far enough, there are always grounds for optimism. Zoom out too far and optimism blurs out human misery in the close folds of history. There is no single vantage point where the perspective is exactly right and no way of knowing where present turmoil fits into a wider story. We can't say how far into the storm we have sailed until the waters are calmer again.

To assert that things will probably turn out better than feared is not to forecast the imminent return of good times, but simply to note that fears for the survival of liberal democracy are calibrated to the absolute worst-case scenario, and by definition, those are less probable than other outcomes.

If it seems, in drawing these conclusions, that I lurch unsteadily between optimism and pessimism, it is because I do. I am not naturally disposed to look on the political bright side. That instinct is compounded by the guilty feeling that complacent liberals were accomplices to the drowning of centrist politics in the rising populist tide. We don't want to repeat the error by predicting that the tide will go out again, revealing our lost Atlantis conveniently preserved by the retreating waters.

Unrealistic optimism is a form of denial, but unremitting pessimism is a self-fulfilling prophecy. If we lean into dread of the abyss, we risk flattering mundanely bad politics by casting it as evil. We empower political fools and petty crooks by thinking they are exceptionally skilled at public manipulation or uniquely persuasive, when their main advantage might simply have been greater motivation and lucky timing.

I have described in this book the systems at work in our politics that exacerbate division, stoke fury and drive reasonable people to seek sanctuary in a state of inner exile. I promised also some prescription for staying engaged without getting enraged. It is an essential task, because the repulsion of an engaged audience – the inducement of hopelessness and doubt that Britain will be governed better – gives succour to those who would make politics worse.

The rage is toxic, but it is not all accidental spill or by-product. A portion is manufactured and the rest exploited to keep politics in a state of febrile frenzy, where rationality and moderation are less competitive. Some of it is made to cynical design by people whose only principle is the acquisition of power. Some of it is ideological stupefaction by politicians who squander resources and talent on the futile business of trying to make reality correspond to nationalist mythology. Often those are the same people at different stages of a journey. The road to self-serving corruption is paved with utopian intention.

There is a risk of falling into the conspiracy theorists' fallacy (observed in Chapter 9), mistaking colossal ineptitude for an ingenious plot, as if the sheer scale of a mess proves it must be intentional. Here, too, lurks a paradox of vigilance – compulsive alertness to deviations from the ideal democracy shade into the paranoid conviction that politics has left the democratic road altogether. A sinister destination is more likely to be reached when enough people think we are there already.

A recurrent theme of this book has been the need for balance and perspective, which involves the more subtle art of keeping balance itself in perspective – holding divergent ideas simultaneously, recognizing that apparently opposing views can both contain *some* truth, but without surrendering to the post-truth relativism that defines a fact as whichever proposition gets the loudest cheer from the biggest mob.

This is the hard kernel of the challenge when populism gains an electoral purchase on democracy. The principled democrat, recognizing the importance of losers' consent to the legitimacy of the system, accepts the popular verdict even when it empowers candidates who don't honour their side of the democratic contract. But what if that victory is bought with flagrant falsehood?

A minority that has irrefutable facts on its side does not become wrong by being outvoted. But it will stay outvoted if it refuses to engage with the reasons for its defeat. Anti-populists do themselves no favours with pious disdain for the voters who cause their misery. They risk becoming the very thing their critics like to accuse them of being: arrogant, elitist and impatient with democracy when it doesn't go their way. By they, I mean we. I mean me.

There is a grey zone between determination never to appease enemies of democracy and a duty of empathy with people who are turning against democracy because it has stopped delivering on its implied promises. It is possible, I believe, and essential to understand the appeal of illiberal and anti-democratic politics without making excuses for its most intolerant expressions or pretending that its elected champions are anything other than dangerous.

One more paradox: the supreme benefit of democracy is that it resolves social conflict without violence, but the argument that it is better than any other system has historically been won by force. Its healthy function requires a critical mass of people who will stay engaged through the times of dysfunction. We endure frustration and disappointment, recognizing that those feelings don't necessarily indicate *systemic* failure of representation. Sometimes we have to endure periods when the views opposing ours are better represented, while keeping faith that our time will come again, arguing, debating, fighting to hasten that moment, but also listening and understanding. The demands of conviction and empathy can pull in conflicting directions. That can be disorienting as we feel our way from fear to hope, treading the line between reasonable vigilance and irrational dread.

Our guide is confidence that no model superior to liberal democracy has been devised, that the alternatives fail, that furious falsehood burns itself out in futile assault on fact. In holding fast to that truth, the supporters of tolerance and pluralism have the resilience to outlast their enemies.

This book is an assertion of that confidence, even if it has sometimes seemed gloomy or dwelled on what look like intractable problems. I don't have a set of technical prescriptions for reform or a bullet-pointed manifesto for a fantasy party of liberal moderation. The task I set myself was diagnostic and therapeutic – to get some critical distance in order to reach a better understanding of what is broken and what can be remedied in our politics; not to conjure false hope that the permacrisis will soon be resolved, but to practise living with volatility. That isn't a counsel of passivity. Actually, the opposite.

I wanted to check that our politics, while often depressing, could still reward civil participation.

British democracy has many flaws, but it isn't a sham. It will become one faster in the duplicitous hands of revolutionary arsonists who preach renewal by means of institutional incineration. Complacency is dangerous, but there is also a hazard in oversteering away from the centre, swerving in hot pursuit of white-knuckle radicals to the left and the right who despise incremental reform and dismiss moderate improvement as tantamount to none. For them the destination is less important than the thrill of the ride.

There are regimes so rotten that the very act of voting is a form of complicity with injustice. Then the only ethical options are to fight or flee. There are conditions where politics is so divorced from sanity that reason can only be cultivated in exile. At the start of this decade, in the darkest moments, I feared Britain was heading in that direction, but I didn't believe the course was predestined. In political debate, reason and tolerance were too often drowned in a bilious cacophony, but I was never persuaded that the noisiest voices spoke for the majority.

I wrote this book in part to redress that imbalance, because I am lucky enough, by virtue of my position as a journalist, to have a voice in political debate. I would have made a terrible politician even before cardiac weakness ruled it out as a practical option. Talking, listening, reading and writing about politics are all I know. With those tools I have tried to illuminate the condition of our democracy and to make what reassurance I might find there contagious.

I have often found comfort in stories that illuminate the character of a problem. It is consoling to discover my perception of things reflected in another mind; not just reflected, but clarified, analyzed and organized. That is how I know I am not alone and not going mad. A crisis can feel less overwhelming when its component parts are laid out neatly on the page. Mental stress is eased by verbal articulation. That isn't to claim that writing is a substitute for action. Nor do I want to defuse anger with analysis in order to somehow anaesthetize demands for change. I would urge anyone who feels passionate about politics to participate as fully as time and temperament allow. Join a party; sign up to a cause; go on a demonstration; deliver leaflets; share facts. (And vote. Always vote.)

But I can't preach what I don't practise. Much though I admire the energies of activists and joiners, envy them even, I am content more often to watch from the sidelines, taking notes.

There is a soothing power in the connection I feel when some writer expresses an idea or feeling that exists somewhere unformed in my mind. The knowledge becomes accessible only once its outline has been crisply drawn in words. The click of association in those moments is a kind of release.

The limit of my ambition for this book is to perform that service for others, or get as close as I can. Is that a political goal or just a journalist's vanity? Does it set the bar too high or too low? I can't judge. Perhaps you were looking for a list of practical tips for a less infuriating democracy. Some thoughts on political self-care are in the epilogue. But anyone reading this far has already demonstrated that, like me, they couldn't just forget about politics and walk away even if they wanted to.

Making explicit the relationship between reader and writer, you and me, is not a marginal part of the argument in this book. It is the reason the book exists. The guide to surviving politics consists in making as many of those connections with as many people as possible.

We carry on reading, writing, talking, sharing through the grim times. We feel the rage but do not surrender to it or let it deactivate our reason. Our anger at the state of politics is proof that we have not given up hope of something better. Fear that we are sliding down to an abyss contains the indomitable will to resist, which history tells us is also a ledge from which we can climb.

That is why I started this chapter from the darkest of all places, in the field of Oświęcim with the teeth that survived the furnace. The men who buried them in the soil had no obvious cause for optimism. Still they imagined a world in which the seeds of truth they planted might become a harvest of remembrance. More than seven decades later, here I am writing about them. And here you are reading about them.

EPILOGUE

REHAB

I get angry about things, then go on and work

Toni Morrison

(i) Coming home

In the first weeks after being discharged from hospital, I had to rest a lot during the day. I was still in a state of heart failure. I was shown the scar on an ultrasound scan, a burned-out strip of flesh where the muscle had died from lack of oxygen. It jerked limply while the surrounding heart pulsed in fleshy undulations.

I spent a few hours each day floating on the edge of wakefulness, and in that half-conscious state, I found a new capacity for lucid recall. I could visit scenes from my past in exquisite detail. I wondered if it was a side effect of medication or the general shock to my system. Either way, it was almost hallucinogenic and not unpleasant. I couldn't replay whole scenes from my youth, but I was able to transport myself back to old places – only interiors. I could feel the contours of the Artex on the walls of my childhood home in the late seventies. I could smell the damp on the charcoal-coloured carpet in the living room of the flat I rented with friends when I left university.

I could explore these spaces with fingertip precision, inch by inch. I remembered the angles of door handles and the action on light switches.

I told my wife that I had emerged from my ordeal with a superpower, albeit not a very practical one. She wasn't impressed. I hoped my extrasensory gift would be permanent, but it faded after a few weeks. I understood it better after it was gone. My hyper-vivid memory had taken me to places I had called home at various stages in life. It was an expression of relief; security. I was reaching out to the past to confirm that it joined up with the present and contained a bridge to a future. I had made it.

Once my heart was strong enough to motor me up and down stairs, I enrolled on a course of cardiac rehabilitation. There were twice-weekly sessions in a local leisure centre. Around 20 of us, almost all men, none younger than me, met to learn more about our condition, how to mend our bodies and our ways.

It reminded me of the driver speed awareness course I once took after being caught on camera driving at 40 mph in a 30 mph zone. There was the same chastened schoolboy vibe. We had broken the cardiac highway code and needed remedial instruction in how to navigate our lives more carefully. There were lectures on what to eat, or rather what not to eat. The basic rule: delicious things are forbidden, except perhaps as occasional treats. 'That means once or twice per week. Not per day,' the instructor clarified.

There was an educational video on what to do in various medical emergencies. Actors bandaged each other's gashed arms, administered Heimlich manoeuvres to dislodge nuts from each other's windpipes, pumped each other's breastplates to restart stalled hearts.

One week, there was a coy film to reassure us that it was safe for cardiac patients to have sex. The excitement wouldn't do us any harm, we were told. 'Most people have a rather exaggerated idea of how much physical exertion is involved,' said the on-screen doctor. No one dissented.

There was a talk on the various pharmaceuticals we were taking and a session on managing stress. I learned how physical symptoms and emotional reactions stoke each other in a feed-back loop. Anxiety accelerates the pulse and causes the release of adrenaline and cortisol – hormones associated with the primal fight-or-flight instinct that tell our brains we are under attack. Once that state is activated, it is much harder to engage analytical and contemplative thought processes. Panic shuts down the slower thinking mode required for cool judgement. Under stress, we make rash decisions that make the stressful situation worse.

I thought about the writhing emotional frenzy I had been in for the years leading up to the heart attack. I remembered the darkening sky. I could picture the hours between feeling the first detonation in my chest and the rush of relief when the stents were inserted as a portal between two dimensions. I had crawled through, just in time. I didn't fancy going back.

The second half of each rehab session, my favourite bit, was supervised exercise. We had our blood pressure taken and heart monitors strapped to our chests. We moved around a dance studio doing various basic aerobic steps – lifting legs, flinging arms, lunging, squatting. We were given target beats-per-minute rates to reach and sustain, but not exceed. I had forgotten what exercise was supposed to feel like. It had been a long time since I had broken a sweat without also feeling a vice closing on my sternum.

It was a fitness class with a hint of prison-yard exercise session. We trooped round in a loop, exchanging the backstories that had landed us in our shared confinement. Some people had been diagnosed with angina after experiencing symptoms like the ones I had ignored for years. There were a lot of mild heart attacks – people who had felt a bit peculiar, mistaken it for indigestion, gone to bed and only decided to visit a hospital when the pain refused to subside. Their arterial obstructions were on the right side of the heart (right as in not left, but also the safer side to have a heart attack, if you're going to have one at all).

Hearing these stories, I felt a perverse pride in my widow-maker, the way a surfer might find affection for the jagged scar that proves survival of a shark attack.

My story was trumped by a guy who'd also had a left coronary artery obstruction but a slower journey to the hospital. He went into ventricular fibrillation in the middle of his angioplasty and had to be jolted back to life with the electric paddles. 'The lights went out,' he said, then paused. 'I get a bit emotional talking about it. Then I was back in the room.' No floating down tunnels towards angelic voices. Just oblivion and reprieve. I remembered my own surgeon's comment when I had pleaded for a pause before the second stent.

'Time is very much of the essence here, Mr Behr.'

Once I got the hang of exercise without chest pain, I started working on politics without fury. I had imposed a news blackout on myself for the first few weeks and had mixed feelings about lifting the embargo. I recognized that I couldn't block the world out forever, but I needed to find new modes of interaction with it. Was there a way to swim in the stream without being swept up in the tide?

Strong emotion could still trigger cardiac discomfort. I went to watch one of my daughters play a football match, a regional cup final. They lost on penalties. I couldn't stay in the arena long enough to see the climax. The adrenaline sent ripples of pain across my chest, chasing the breath out of my lungs.

I worried that turning up in Westminster would do something similar, and that I would need to find something different to write about for a living. But I didn't know enough about anything other than politics.

One Wednesday lunchtime, I experimented with watching a few minutes of Prime Minister's Questions live from the House of Commons. I was reassured to find that Boris Johnson's bloviation didn't interfere with my mental composure or my breathing. I was struck above all by the smallness of the spectacle. It seemed like a sign that Britain had failed to take itself seriously as a country, and although I found that dispiriting, I was not incapacitated by rage. It would be wrong to say that I cared less. I cared differently.

(ii) Slowing down

I stopped eating junk. I lost around 10 kilos. I found I could fit back into the suit I wore on my wedding day. In the early weeks I wasn't even tempted by pastries and chocolate, which had been my weakness before the heart attack. A prickly shadow still stroked my ribs from time to time, gently invigilating dietary discipline.

Recalling the old emotional agitation helped enforce abstinence from social media. I knew I would have to go back one day. Digital platforms are hard-wired into the political operating system. To ignore them would be to miss part of the Westminster picture, but I was in no hurry to restart my old habit.

I adopted pretty much the same rules for consuming information as I applied to the saturated fat, sugar and salt in my meals. I found it useful to think of the effects as analogous. Junk food clogs your arteries, sends your blood pressure up and makes you fat; junk news causes political hypertension, cognitive cholesterol, flabby thinking. Scrolling through the sources that tell us what we want to hear, we sink into the comfy sofa of our prejudices, lounging in the greasy pyjamas of self-righteous affirmation.

Unlike a newspaper or magazine, the internet has no last page. There is no natural end point to the digital browsing session. We pluck out our phones for some task, and before we can even remember what it was, our attention is grabbed by a passing notification. We are once again reaching into the bottomless Pringles tube of refined info-mulch. The binge stops either when something in the analogue world demands our attention or when we are checked by a spasm of disgust at the amount of time wasted feasting on empty news calories.

It is an addiction. For the first few days, not looking at a phone felt very much like the experience of trying (and often failing) to quit smoking. There was the same restlessness, the same twitchiness in the hands bereft of something to hold, the same feeling of being stalked by an absence.

Nicotine activates receptors in the brain that release dopamine – a potent feel-good chemical that gets involved whenever you do something pleasurable. It is there when you eat delicious food, wake from a good night's sleep, score a goal, have sex. The insidious genius of the cigarette is the way it mimics the gratification of getting things done. It whispers success in your mind's ear. The first few drags send out a tingle of reward for having accomplished something. By lighting a cigarette, you have indeed solved a problem – the problem of not having a lit cigarette in your mouth.

Social media plays on the same cycle of false reward and renewed craving. Journalists love Twitter because it seems to satisfy two appetites that come with the job – compulsion to know what is happening and the need for an audience. Having your own tweets liked and shared generates a hit of recognition. Even hostile reaction feeds the addiction, either because you feel obliged to defend yourself or because you don't want to log out on a negative note. You have a bitter taste in your mouth after reading abuse, and kid yourself that more tweeting will rinse it away.

But with sufficient digital hygiene – blocking and muting the lunatics – social media can also be a bountiful source of useful information and illuminating ideas. For every maniacal troll, there are plenty of witty and thoughtful voices. There are people I have never met offline but whose sanity and good humour on the internet has kept me balanced and, by reasonable argument, changed my mind. Not everyone online is bellowing bile. But I don't need a digital chorus to greet me first thing in the morning or accompany me to bed. I switch off at weekends and on holidays.

I rebalanced my news diet. I sought out original reporting, even-tempered analysis supported by wholesome data, sources of information fibre and factual nutrition without the sugar rush of outrage. I focused more on international stories, not because they were uplifting but because the global context brings nuance to Britain's predicament. Paranoia about national decline is accelerated by the parochialism of our news agenda.

Once I stopped doom-scrolling, I became conscious of a change in mental tempo that comes when you no longer interrupt your own thought process with a luminous screen. The search for news had rarely been the real reason for taking my phone out of my pocket. Nine times out of ten, there would be no particular thing I was looking for, no destination, just a vague itch to scratch.

I suspect that the trigger had been unconscious reluctance to let my mind wander by itself, unguided by the algorithm of sequential distractions. How had I become so mentally unadventurous? When had I decided that my train of thought needed derailing before it even left the station? Letting it roll down the track reminded me of being a child, having a space to explore that was virtual but not digital. The word for that realm is imagination.

(iii) Looking up

I don't claim to have reached a Zen state of post-fury. My family would laugh at the idea, especially when I'm on a deadline.

I am also aware how much my peace of mind is a luxury afforded by a steady job and a comfortable income, and how much of survival is arbitrary. A few hundred metres further down the road with a clot forming in the left coronary artery and maybe the way back is too far. Wait too long for an ambulance and maybe there is no electric paddle to bring the lights back on.

Equanimity achieved by way of dumb luck can easily shade into fatalism. Basking in the feeling of a bonus life extension, won by chance, I enjoyed a phase of blithe indifference to politics. But it started to feel irresponsible, not to mention professionally limiting. I had to care enough to want to write. And when politics degrades the country you call home there is a responsibility to stay angry in defiance of those who seek to gain from disengagement.

But these days I approach that duty with a question. What portion of the anger is organically mine and how much is synthetic? Some of it is a poisonous substance sprayed out by the machinery that I have to operate and the company I must keep for work. There is a method for handling that compound. I decant it carefully onto the page with less spillage into the rest of my life.

I have an old notebook where I used to copy out quotes from books that I admired. I forgot about it for years. Leafing through it recently, I found a line spoken by a character in a Philip Roth novel, *I Married a Communist*: 'Anger is to make you effective. That's its survival function. That's why it's given to you. If it makes you ineffective, drop it like a hot potato.'

Outrage is not inherently toxic to democracy. It can be the necessary antidote to apathy, but it also has to be the spur to something else. It has to lead somewhere that isn't just more rage.

The emotional root of anger is fear. It is a defensive reaction against perceived threat. I am better now at seeing the hostility in other people – and myself – as an expression of anxiety and insecurity. Whether on social media or in real life, incivility and aggression spring from dread of losing control. In politics, they arise when someone feels under attack, which is an increasingly common reaction in any argument where the boundaries between partisan opinion, public policy and personal identity are blurred.

People do not respond kindly to views that they experience as an injury to their sacred beliefs. That response might not be rational, but the feeling is real, and telling someone to get over it doesn't help. The trick is not to take it personally, even when it *is* personal.

The Hungarian mathematician George Pólya had good advice for anyone overwhelmed by a complex challenge: 'If you can't solve a problem, then there is an easier problem you can solve: find it.' It doesn't apply exactly in politics, because mathematical problems tend to have precise solutions. The equation can be simplified. A graph can be plotted and the answer found at the exact place where the lines cross. Maths abhors grey areas. But there is still a political application for Pólya's principle of locating the doable part of a problem. In apparently intractable, polarized arguments, there is nearly always a place of common understanding somewhere – some sliver of terrain where the terms of reality are mutually recognizable. Find that; build on it.

After nearly two years as a cardiac outpatient, I was given the all-clear in the spring of 2022. First I had to submit to something called a nuclear stress test, which sounded like the sort of thing that should be done in a concrete bunker underneath an American desert. In reality, it meant going to a hospital, swallowing a radioactive isotope that illuminates the arterial routes carrying blood to the heart, taking a drug that excites the cardiovascular system and lying under an MRI machine that can locate any blockages.

I was offered a blanket. Then I remembered that the room needed to be kept at a fridge-like temperature to protect the scanning machines. I remembered how violently I had shivered during my emergency angioplasty. I remembered wondering if that was what was meant by a 'death rattle' – if the doctors were holding me down to prevent me shuffling off the mortal coil. It turns out I was just cold.

The isotope found no sneaky obstructions building in the back roads behind my heart. Ingesting a toxin in controlled conditions, managed correctly, could be illuminating, I thought.

The doctor offered reassurance that the procedure would leave me only mildly radioactive, although a leaflet I had been given warned against hugging children for at least 24 hours. With that proviso, I was discharged; good to go.

I had already bought myself a heart-rate monitor and started running again. I built up the pace and distance slowly. For the first few outings, I avoided the route I had taken on New Year's Eve 2019. The first time I went that way, I passed the exact spot where my heart had malfunctioned and carried on through, reaching the park with tears in my eyes. Then it became part of my regular itinerary. I still put on an extra burst of speed when I get to that corner, leaping over the ghost of myself lying on the pavement, giving thanks to the ghost of Eliyahu Rinkunsky.

I go up to the South Downs or along the Brighton seashore, anywhere that affords a distant horizon. There is a technique to distance running that I had not known before. You need to check for hazards at your feet, but mostly keep your head up and your shoulders back, unclench your fists. Look out, look up. That is how I keep things in perspective, especially when the anger rises and I need to think my way through it, to run through it, until I have reached the other side and found my way home.

BIBLIOGRAPHY

Listed here are works that are mentioned or quoted in the text, plus a selection that I read (or in some cases reread) while writing this book and that had some influence on its direction.

Aaronovitch, David, *Voodoo Histories: How conspiracy theory has shaped modern history*, Vintage, 2010

Applebaum, Anne, *Twilight of Democracy: The failure of politics and the parting of friends*, Allen Lane, 2020

Arendt, Hannah, *The Origins of Totalitarianism*, Schocken, 1951

Baddiel, David, *Jews Don't Count*, HarperCollins, 2021

Baldwin, Tom, *Ctrl Alt Delete: How politics and the media crash our democracy*, Hurst, 2018

Collins, Matthew, *Hate: My life in the British far right*, Biteback, 2011

d'Ancona, Matthew, *Identity, Ignorance, Innovation: Why the old politics is useless and what to do about it*, Hodder & Stoughton, 2021

Didion, Joan, *Slouching Towards Bethlehem: Essays*, Farrar, Straus and Giroux, 1968

Duffy, Bobby, *Generations: Does when you're born shape who you are?*, Atlantic, 2021

Dunt, Ian, *How to Be a Liberal*, Canbury, 2022

Eddo-Lodge, Reni, *Why I'm No Longer Talking to White People About Race*, Bloomsbury, 2017

Elledge, Jonn, and Phillips, Tom, *Conspiracy: A history of b*llocks theories and how not to fall for them*, Headline, 2022

Farage, Nigel, *The Purple Revolution: The year that changed everything*, Biteback, 2015

Ferguson, Niall, *Doom: The politics of catastrophe*, Allen Lane, 2021

Freedland, Jonathan, *Jacob's Gift: A journey into the heart of belonging*, Hamish Hamilton, 2005

Fukuyama, Francis, *The End of History and the Last Man*, Free Press, 1992

——*Liberalism and its Discontents*, Profile, 2022

Gardner, Dan, *Future Babble: How to stop worrying and love the unpredictable*, Virgin, 2011

Geoghegan, Peter, *Democracy for Sale: Dark money and dirty politics*, Head of Zeus, 2020

Glaser, Eliane, *Elitism: A progressive defence*, Biteback, 2020

Goffman, Erving, *The Presentation of Self in Everyday Life*, Doubleday, 1959

Goodhart, David, *The Road to Somewhere: The populist revolt and the future of politics*, Hurst & Co., 2017

Grossman, David, *Writing in the Dark*, Bloomsbury 2008

Haidt, Jonathan, *The Righteous Mind: Why good people are divided by politics and religion*, Penguin, 2012

Hardman, Isabel, *Why We Get the Wrong Politicians*, Atlantic, 2018

Harford, Tim, *How to Make the World Add Up*, Bridge Street, 2020

Hawes, James, *The Shortest History of England*, Old Street, 2020

Hawley, Katherine, *Trust: A very short introduction*, Oxford, 2012

Higgs, John, *The Future Starts Here: Adventures in the twenty-first century*, Weidenfeld & Nicolson, 2019

Hosking, George, and Schöpflin, George, *Myths and Nationhood*, Hurst & Co., 1997

Hutton, Robert, *Agent Jack: The true story of MI5's secret Nazi hunter*, Weidenfeld & Nicolson, 2018

Ignatieff, Michael, *Fire and Ashes: Success and failure in politics*, Random House, 2013

James, Clive, *Unreliable Memoirs*, Jonathan Cape, 1980

——*Cultural Amnesia: Notes in the margin of my time*, Picador, 2007

——*The Revolt of the Pendulum: Essays 2005–2008*, Picador, 2009

Judt, Tony, *Reappraisals: Reflections on the forgotten twentieth century*, Vintage, 2009

Kahneman, Daniel, *Thinking, Fast and Slow*, Allen Lane, 2011

Koestler, Arthur, *Scum of the Earth*, Jonathan Cape, 1941

Krastev, Ivan, and Holmes, Stephen, *The Light That Failed: A reckoning*, Allen Lane, 2019

Kundera, Milan, *The Joke*, Faber & Faber, 1969

Kuper, Simon, *Chums: How a tiny caste of Oxford Tories took over the UK*, Profile, 2022

Leslie, Ian, *Conflicted: Why arguments are tearing us apart and how they can bring us together*, Faber & Faber, 2021

Levi, Primo, *If This Is a Man*, 1958

——*The Drowned and the Saved*, 1986

Lewens, Tim, *The Meaning of Science*, Pelican, 2015

Milosz, Czeslaw, *The Captive Mind*, 1953

Mishra, Pankaj, *Age of Anger: A history of the present*, Penguin, 2017

O'Toole, Fintan, *Heroic Failure: Brexit and the politics of pain*, Head of Zeus, 2019

Orwell, George, *Essays*, Penguin, 1984

——*Nineteen Eighty-Four*, 1949

Payne, Sebastian, *Broken Heartlands, A journey through Labour's lost England*, Macmillan, 2021

Peston, Robert, *WTF?*, Hodder & Stoughton, 2017

Pinker, Steven, *Rationality: What it is, why it seems scarce, why it matters*, Penguin, 2021

Pomerantsev, Peter, *This Is Not Propaganda: Adventure in the war against reality*, Faber & Faber, 2019

Prosser, Thomas, *What's in It for Me?: Self-interest and political difference*, Manchester University Press, 2021

Runciman, David, *Politics*, Profile, 2014

——*How Democracy Ends*, Profile, 2018

Sandel, Michael J., *The Tyranny of Merit: What's become of the common good?*, Penguin, 2020

Sanghera, Sathnam, *Empireland: How imperialism has shaped modern Britain*, Penguin, 2021

Shafak, Elif, *How to Stay Sane in an Age of Division*, Profile, 2020

Sharot, Tali, *The Optimism Bias*, Pantheon, 2011

Shipman, Tim, *All Out War: The full story of Brexit*, HarperCollins, 2017

Snyder, Timothy, *On Tyranny: Twenty lessons from the twentieth century*, The Bodley Head, 2017

Temelkuran, Ece, *How to Lose a Country: The seven steps from democracy to dictatorship*, 4th Estate, 2019

Tolentino, Jia, *Trick Mirror: Reflections on self-delusion*, 4th Estate, 2019

Turner, Alwyn, *A Classless Society: Britain in the 1990s*, Aurum, 2013

Walker, Carole, *Lobby Life: Inside Westminster's secret society*, Elliott and Thompson, 2021

Westen, Drew, *The Political Brain: The role of emotion in deciding the fate of the nation*, Public Affairs, 2008

Yates, Jon, *Fractured: Why our societies are coming apart and how we put them back together again*, HarperNorth, 2021

Young, Hugo, *Supping with the Devils: Political writing from Thatcher to Blair*, Atlantic, 2003

ACKNOWLEDGEMENTS

This book would not exist without the cardiology ward of the Royal Sussex County Hospital, and nor would its author. I owe them the first portion of gratitude. An equal measure of thanks goes to the Sussex Heart Charity, whose cardiac rehabilitation classes helped me restart ordinary life before I could think about re-engaging with politics.

To get from an idea for a book to an actual book required encouragement and advice from a number of people. Essential contributions came from Matt d'Ancona, Mike Harpley, Caroline Michel and Richard Charkin. The journey from vague notion to viable project could not have been completed without the energy and focus of Rory Scarfe. The manuscript was much improved by comments from better writers than me. Particular thanks to David Aaronovitch, Helen Lewis, Rob Hutton, Fintan O'Toole, Sathnam Sanghera and Jamie Susskind for reading ragged bits of early drafts, which benefited greatly from their attention. The remaining deficiencies indicate deviation from their advice. Reading at the very last minute is a service for which I am indebted to 'Professor' Michael Philipedes.

The best editors have a knack for guiding writers to the changes they already know, deep down, need making. Ed Faulkner at Atlantic performed that service with great sensitivity and dependable judgement. Jane Selley's expert editorial eye was also crucial.

The *Guardian* has been a hugely supportive employer. For their patience and encouragement, I am grateful to Kath Viner and Jan Thompson; also to Hugh Muir, the opinion desk team and the leader writers in whose erudite company it is a privilege to sit.

Where the book strays into psychology, it channels conversations with guests it has been my good fortune to interview for the *Politics on the Couch* podcast. That wouldn't have been possible without the industry and intellect of Philip Berman, a top producer and friend.

It was probably possible to survive the darkest phases of British politics without the solidarity and lucid intelligence of Jonathan Freedland, but I'm glad I never had to try.

Political journalism often relies on information and insight shared anonymously. I won't breach that contract here, but my sources know who they are. I thank them.

If the importance to this project of my parents and my brother was not made clear enough in the opening chapters, let me emphasize it here, with additional love and gratitude. For fact-checking on scenes from Finchley and Netanya, among other valuable inputs, I credit the eminent co-founder of the SC.

To my wife, Emily, and daughters, Edie and Martha, I record here an apology for the amount of my time and attention consumed by the production of this book. When there were not enough hours in the day, my family did not ration their patience and support. While other resources might be constrained, the inspiration I get from them has no limit.

INDEX